Circumcision - Advances and New Perspectives

Edited by Ahmad Zaghal and Ali El Safadi

Published in London, United Kingdom

Circumcision - Advances and New Perspectives
http://dx.doi.org/10.5772/intechopen.101011
Edited by Ahmad Zaghal and Ali El Safadi

Contributors
Mehmet Uysal, Claudio Militello, Veronica Pais, Giuseppe Saitta, Rosario Leonardi, Rodrigo Garcia-Baquero, Cristina M. Fernández-Ávila, José Luis Álvarez-Ossorio, Ahmad Zaghal, Ali El Safadi

First published in London, United Kingdom, 2023 by IntechOpen
IntechOpen is the global imprint of INTECHOPEN LIMITED, registered in England and Wales, registration number: 11086078, 5 Princes Gate Court, London, SW7 2QJ, United Kingdom

British Library Cataloguing-in-Publication Data
A catalogue record for this book is available from the British Library

Additional hard and PDF copies can be obtained from orders@intechopen.com

Circumcision - Advances and New Perspectives
Edited by Ahmad Zaghal and Ali El Safadi
p. cm.
Print ISBN 978-1-80355-906-3
Online ISBN 978-1-80355-907-0
eBook (PDF) ISBN 978-1-80355-908-7

Meet the editors

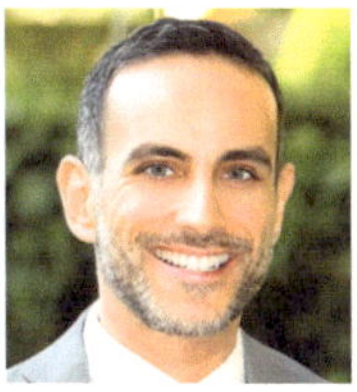

Ahmad Zaghal, MD, MSc (Clin Ed), FACS, FEBPS, graduated from the general surgery residency program at the American University of Beirut Medical Center (AUBMC), Lebanon, in 2012. He then completed a two-year fellowship in pediatric surgery at the University of Iowa Hospitals and Clinics, USA, and a further year of fellowship in the same specialism at Chelsea and Westminster Hospital, UK. He has been a pediatric surgeon and assistant professor of surgery at AUBMC since 2017. Dr. Zaghal is board certified by the European Board of Pediatric Surgery. His special interests are minimally invasive and neonatal surgery, and medical education. He is a fellow of the Higher Education Academy. Dr. Zaghal has published several articles in peer-reviewed journals and authored several chapters in general and pediatric surgery books.

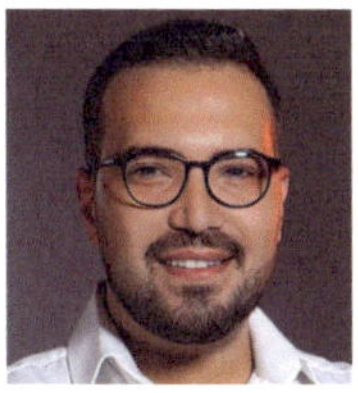

Dr. Ali El Safadi graduated from the School of Medicine, Lebanese American University (LAU), in 2020, and is currently completing his residency training in the Department of Obstetrics and Gynecology at the American University of Beirut Medical Center. Dr. El Safadi is interested in basic and clinical research, with a particular focus on innovation, technology, and medical education. He has authored several articles in peer-reviewed journals and presented his work at national and international conferences.

Contents

Preface

The practice of circumcising males for prophylactic reasons dates back over 6,000 years to ancient Egypt, as well as to cultures, such as in Sub-Saharan Africa, where it was performed on boys as a rite of passage into adulthood.

Today, opinions on circumcision remain divided, with some people opposing it and others investing in programs to circumcise men in regions with high rates of HIV infection. The different circumcision techniques described in the literature include both traditional and innovative methods.

This book helps healthcare providers to familiarize themselves with the different techniques for male circumcision, in order to provide optimal care and the best surgical outcomes for those seeking the procedure.

Ahmad Zaghal, MD, MSc (Clin Ed), FACS, FEBPS
Department of General Surgery,
American University of Beirut Medical Center,
Beirut, Lebanon

Ali El Safadi, MD
Department of Obstetrics and Gynecology,
American University of Beirut Medical Center,
Beirut, Lebanon

Section 1

Introduction

Chapter 1

Introductory Chapter: Novelty Meets Tradition

Ahmad Zaghal and Ali El Safadi

1. Introduction

Male circumcision has been practiced for centuries by different cultures; nowadays, it is considered one of the most commonly performed surgical procedures worldwide. The oldest picture depicting circumcision dates back to 2300 BC in ancient Egypt; it was considered a symbol of pledge between God and Abraham [1].

Apart from cultural and religious perspectives, circumcision is performed for medical reasons including preventing sexually transmitted diseases, recurrent urinary tract infections, phimosis, and balanoposthitis [2]. In 2007, the World Health Organization (WHO) recommended the practice of youth and adult circumcision as an effective method to prevent the transmission of Human Immunodeficiency virus (HIV) in high endemic areas [3].

There are different circumcision techniques described in the literature. The WHO manual on male circumcision recommends mainly three adult and four pediatric techniques for circumcision. The sleeve resection, surgical dorsal slit, and forceps-guided are advised for adults, whereas the Plastibell method, Mogen and Gomco clamps, and the dorsal slit technique are advised for the pediatric population [4].

2. Novel techniques for male circumcision

Currently, circumcision is performed using different techniques depending on instruments availability and surgeons' expertise. Most commonly utilized circumcision methods include Gomco clamp, Mogen clamp, Plastibell, dorsal slit, and bone cutter. Ring circumcision devices such as Plastibell, Shang Ring, and other plastic rings are popular and are the preferred instruments for circumcision due to their ease of usage, they allow a less traumatic technique with a low complication rate and better cosmetic outcomes [5].

Advances in the medical field have brought into light new methods to perform male circumcision. These techniques permit more desirable clinical outcomes in terms of less morbidity for the patient, less to no pain, shorter procedural time, and better cosmetic outcomes.

Laser circumcision (LC) has recently received attention as one of the innovative techniques of circumcision. A high-intensity light beam is used to cut and seal the foreskin. There are various types of LC namely using heat, carbon dioxide, or neodymium as energy output. Neodymium: yttrium-aluminum-garnet (Nd-YAG) lasers permit accurate cutting while achieving hemostasis and minimal tissue damage [6].

IntechOpen

Carbon dioxide laser beam is used in focused mode to resect a demarcated circumferential incision through the skin reaching the subcutaneous mucosa. Because of its thermocoagulation effect, hemostasis is reached by cauterizing the small blood vessels with surrounding tissue [7].

Heat energy Metzenbaum scissors can be used as an alternative to conventional clamps in which circumcision is performed using bipolar scissors to remove the foreskin and underlying mucosa and proceed with the frenulotomy, and then closure of the wound is achieved using synthetic sutures depending on the size and age of the patient [8].

3. Comparable overview of various techniques used in circumcision

After circumcision, the penis is inspected for possible lacerations, bleeding, inflammation, hematoma, and edema. There are various factors that dictate potential acute complications including anatomical variances, patient's age, and surgical technique used.

Studies exploring complication rates of circumcision are sparse, but available statistics denote the overall complication rate of this procedure between 0.2 and 5% [9].

Traditional techniques such as dorsal slits and forceps-guided methods require more surgical expertise and procedural time than other traditional methods like Mogen and Gomco clamps, and Plastibell, which require shorter surgical time. Furthermore, they are easy to learn and perform. Less cosmetic satisfaction was noted using the dorsal slit method because of lack of symmetrical foreskin cutting [10].

Comparing the Mogen clamp and Plastibell method, studies have shown more risk of nonstandard amputation of the glans penis with the Mogen clamp, whereas Plastibell displacement can cause glans necrosis. However, higher risk of lacerations and bleeding was seen with Gomco clamp usage [11, 12].

The most common acute complication with the use of Plastibell is bleeding with a rate ranging between 2.5 and 4%. Paraphimosis is another complication of Plastibell technique attributed to the dislodgement of the plastic ring [13, 14].

The use of bipolar scissors for foreskin cutting in circumcision is comparatively new. Marsh et al. reported the first case of bipolar usage in 1995 [15]. Common acute complications of this procedure include bleeding, edema, erythema, hematoma, and pain [8].

Carbon dioxide laser-directed circumcision has been shown to provide adequate incision and hemostatic properties under the effect of small vessel cauterization. In addition, better cosmetic outcomes were noted with the use of laser and less postoperative pain compared to the conventional scalpel method [7].

4. Future perspectives

Male circumcision can be safely performed at any age, but most of the procedures are done during infancy. That said, most of the procedures are done at an early age to maximize circumcision benefits and reduce possible adverse events [16]. Various techniques are used to perform male circumcision. When performed properly, surgical complications rate is low. Minor complications are noted between 0.5 and 1% when performed in infancy [17].

Current studies are directed at describing a technique that can achieve the best surgical and cosmetic outcomes for the patient and attempt to prevent transmission of HIV [18]. Traditional and novel techniques for circumcision are detailed in the literature in terms of proper usage, pros and cons of each technique, and efficacy of innovative methods compared to traditional ones. Few new techniques of circumcision are described in the literature, however, there is not enough data to compare their efficacy and safety profiles with the traditional methods, and hence they are not yet fully supported.

It is key for the healthcare providers to acquaint themselves with available procedures for male circumcision that can potentially deliver the optimal care and best surgical outcomes for boys and men seeking circumcision.

Author details

Ahmad Zaghal* and Ali El Safadi
Department of Surgery, American University of Beirut Medical Center, Lebanon

*Address all correspondence to: az22@aub.edu.lb

References

[1] Meijer B, Butzelaar RM. Circumcisie in historisch perspectief [Circumcision from a historical perspective]. Ned Tijdschr Geneeskd. 2000;**144**(52):2504-2508

[2] Anwer AW, Samad L, Iftikhar S, Baig-Ansari N. Reported male circumcision practices in a muslim-majority setting. BioMed Research International. 2017;**2017**:4957348

[3] WHO. Preventing HIV through Safe Voluntary Medical Male Circumcision for Adolescent Boys and Men in Generalized HIV Epidemics. Geneva, Switzerland: World Health Organization; 2020

[4] Hargreave T. Male circumcision: Towards a World Health Organisation normative practice in resource limited settings. Asian Journal of Andrology. 2010;**12**(5):628-638

[5] WHO/UNAIDS. Male Circumcision: Global Trends and Determinants of Prevalence, Safety, and Acceptability. Geneva, Switzerland: World Health Organization; 2008

[6] Xu Y, Li F, Li Z, et al. A prospective, randomized controlled trial of circumcision in adult males using the CO_2 laser: Modified technique compared with the conventional dorsal-slit technique. Photomed Laser Surgery. 2013;**31**:422-427

[7] Ronchi P, Manno S, Dell'Atti L. Technology meets tradition: CO_2 laser circumcision versus conventional surgical technique. Research and Reports in Urology. 2020;**12**:255

[8] Méndez-Gallart R, et al. Bipolar scissors circumcision is a safe, fast, and bloodless procedure in children. Journal of Pediatric Surgery. 2009;**44**(10):2048-2053

[9] Kaplan GW. Complications of circumcision. Urology Clinical North America. 1983;**10**:543-546

[10] Lei JH, Liu LR, Wei Q, et al. Circumcision with "no-flip Shang Ring" and "Dorsal Slit" methods for adult males: A single-centered, prospective, clinical study. Asian Journal of Andrology. 2016;**18**(5):798-802

[11] Plank RM, Ndubuka NO, Wirth KE, et al. A randomized trial of Mogen clamp versus Plastibell for neonatal male circumcision in Bostwana. Journal of Acquired Immune Deficiency Syndrome. 2013;**62**(5):e131-e137

[12] Chan PS, Penna FJ, Holmes AV. Gomco versus Mogen? No effect on circumcision revision rates. Hospial Pediatric. 2018;**8**(10):611-614

[13] Bastos JM, Netto G, de Araújo J, Jr NMF, Passos BR, Lopes HE, et al. A prospective evaluation of Plastibell® circumcision in older children. International Brazil Journal of Urology. 2013;**39**(4):558-564

[14] Al-Ghazo MA, Banihani KE. Circumcision revision in male children. International Brazil Journal of Urology. 2006;**32**(4):454-458

[15] Marsh SK, Archer TJ. Bipolar diathermy haemostasis during circumcision. Journal of British Surgery. 1995;**82**(4):533

[16] Blank S, Brady M, Buerk E, Carlo W, Diekema D, Freedman A, et al. American academy of pediatrics, task force on circumcision: Male circumcision. Pediatrics. 2012;**130**:e756-e785

[17] Weiss HA, Larke N, Halperin D, Schenker I. Complications of circumcision in male neonates, infants and children: A systematic review. BMC Urology. 2010;**10**:2

[18] Mutabazi V, Kaplan SA, Rwamasirabo E, Bitega JP, Ngeruka ML, Savio D, et al. HIV prevention: Male circumcision comparison between a nonsurgical device to a surgical technique in resource-limited settings: A prospective, randomized, nonmasked trial. Journal of Acquired Immune Deficiency Syndrome. 2012;**61**:49-55

Section 2

Circumcision Techniques

Chapter 2

Male Circumcision: History of Current Surgical Practice

Claudio Militello and Veronica Pais

Abstract

One of the most frequent procedures carried out on men, whether for medical or religious reasons, is circumcision, which involves the removal of the foreskin. The procedure's introduction in various locations and times allowed for the development of a surgical approach that is now adapted to minimize problems and deliver obvious medicinal benefits. Male circumcision is currently a hot topic of dispute because of ethical, legal, and scientific concerns, as well as the procedure's various roles: therapeutic, preventive, and ritualistic. The practice's origins can be traced back to ancient times, but it is still a surgical procedure used to prevent HIV transmission today. In order to lower the risk of HIV transmission in men, the WHO advised considering male circumcision in 2007. The purpose of this article is to describe the procedure of circumcision throughout history.

Keywords: circumcision, history, religious, ritual, techniques

1. Introduction

Male circumcision is one of the maximum carried out surgical methods withinside the world. The surgical treatment for correction of phimosis, the narrowness of the hole of the foreskin that stops overall or partial uncovering of the glans., is given numerous names. From the Latin circum (around) and caedere (to reduce) [1], to the partial or overall excision of the foreskin; in scientific nomenclature, it has the denominations of postectomy (from the Greek: posthé - prepuce; ektomé - resection), postoplasty (from the Greek: plastes or plastic - that forms), or the mixture of both, postectoplasty [2].

It is one of the oldest surgical strategies known, historically undertaken as a mark of cultural identity or religion. With advances in surgical operation withinside the nineteenth century and withinside the twentieth century, the method changed into delivered into a few formerly non-circumcising cultures for each health-associated and social reasons [3].

As of 2016, the worldwide incidence of circumcision is envisioned to be around 38% [4]; due to this high percentage, World Health Organization and UNAIDS have promoted better use of circumcision in nations with a high prevalence of HIV as prophylaxis to this disease [3].

The objective of this publication is to conduct a narrative review of the circumcision procedure during history.

2. Circumcision from a historical perspective

2.1 Circumcision in the ancient age

Regarding the origins of circumcision, anthropologists disagree. Sir Crafton Elliot Smith, an English Egyptologist, argued that it is one of the traits of a society known as the "heliolithic," which originated in Egypt and expanded throughout most of the world around 15,000 years ago, according to Dunsmuir and Gordon [5].

The proof that favors the idea that circumcision started withinside the Heliolithic tradition in Ancient Egypt is documented in a papyrus so-known as Ebers Papyrus, discovered in Luxor in 1862 by the German archeologist Georg Moritz Ebers (1837–1898) discovered among the legs of a mummy in Thebes and dated to 3000 B.C; the text included step-by-step directions for executing the procedure [1]. The topic of whether Egyptians circumcised their males as a religious ritual or as a surgical procedure for hygiene purposes is intriguing. It appears that Egyptian circumcision was performed as a preventative hygienic measure to ensure excellent sanitation of the balano-preputial groove; this makes sense because the Ebers Papyrus is one of the oldest known medical and pharmacopeia treatises [1]. However, it does not appear that the practice was wholly devoid of ritual implications, as it was once restricted to priests, aristocrats, and members of the royal family [1].

Several authors [1, 3–10] described another relic that shows that Egyptians practiced circumcision and was discovered in Saqqarah, Egypt, in the entryway of the tomb of the sixth dynasty pharaoh Ankhmahor, which represented a circumcision scene (**Figure 1**). This relic dates back to King Teti's reign (2355–2343 B.C.).

Totaro et al. [1] referred that the Chaldeans, a polytheistic Semitic tribe who settled in southern Mesopotamia in the early part of the 1st millennium B.C, also knew of circumcision in the mountains of Armenia and Kurdistan, as documented in clay tablets found in 1849 in the ruins of the Royal Palace of Nineveh. These tablets were believed to have been produced in 1600 B.C [1].

The Israelites were another Middle Eastern society that used circumcision. Regarding circumcision, some authors [1, 5–7, 11] indicated that it dates back to Abraham's prophet, while others, such as Herodotus (a Greek historian and geographer), have stated that it was brought to Egypt by the Israelites during their captivity circa 1200 BC. It is interesting to comment that the circumcision agreed upon by the Jews could have been interrupted in the year 169 before Christ. Doyle (6 pp280–281) wrote out that Antiochus IV Epiphanes (king of Syria of the Seleucid dynasty from around 175 BC–164 BC), besieged Jerusalem in 169 BC, quartered his troops inside the temple, and declared the circumcision to be unlawful and temporarily abolished the practice.

Circumcision was also practiced in ancient Rome. This is justified by what was published in the medical treatise written by Aulus Cornelius Celsus (25 B.C-50 A.D) where it was explained that given the impossibility of exposing the glans, the skin that covers it should be surgically opened [1].

In 660 A.D., Muslims practiced circumcision. Despite the fact that the Quran does not mention circumcision by name, it has come to be seen as an essential component of that faith [1, 6].

2.2 Circumcision in the middle ages

In the Middle Ages, an outstanding Italian surgeon, Theodoric Borgognoni, in his book published in 1267 and called "Theodoric's Surgery", recommended that in order

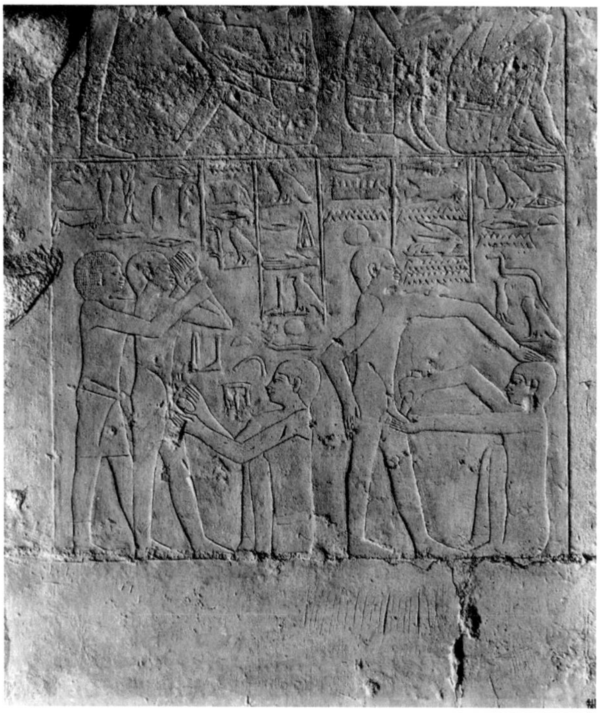

Figure 1.
Egyptian wall carving showing a circumcision scene, Sakkara. Wellcome collection. Attribution 4.0 international (CC BY 4.0). Public domain mark.

to treat certain penile diseases such as warts and tubercles, "the last component of the penis should be removed". It is believed that this author was describing circumcision as a treatment for certain diseases of the penis [5]. The French surgeon Guy de Chauliac (1360 AD) referred to the fact that circumcision in this period was performed to prevent the accumulation of dirt at the base of the glans. Another medieval Ottoman surgeon Serefeddin Sabuncuoglu (1385–1470 AD) offers one of the earliest descriptions of Muslim circumcision [5].

2.3 Circumcision in the modern and contemporary age

Early in the 19th century, textbooks start to include brief explanations of adult circumcision for phimosis. Dr. John Abernethy recounts using the scalpel (knife) to perform circumcision on men with "gonococcal" in 1828, despite the fact that surgical techniques are rarely reported in detail. Additionally, he said that any bleeding must be "sealed with iodoform and boric," which may mean that no sutures were used [5].

The appearance of circumcision for medical reasons dates to the mid-19th century. This increase can be attributed to two events. First, within Victorian thought, everything that had to do with sexuality was considered sinful. According to this, masturbation was seen as the cause of many diseases. As physicians in the second half of the 19th century believed that circumcision would prevent masturbation, circumcision spread rapidly during that period, particularly in the Anglo-American world. Second, surgical treatments were attempted for many ailments at the time, after all, the real cause was unknown [9].

The first circumcision reported [5] in surgical accounts from St Bartholomew's Hospital was in 1865. One of the staunchest advocates of circumcision for medical reasons was the American physician PC Remondino [9, 10]. In his 1891 book, "A History of Circumcision," circumcision is described as a measure to prevent or cure many diverse ailments [5, 9, 10, 12], including alcoholism, syphilis, epilepsy, inguinal hernia, and asthma. Remondino's views are well illustrated by his comment: "It really seems that the foreskin is always a dangerous risk, and life insurance companies may classify the use of a foreskin under the heading of dangerous risks" [9].

The change from the 19th to the 20th century was also an important moment to lay the foundations of the surgical technique. Sir Frederick Treves (1903) gives us a complete description of the basic surgical principles that are maintained today. In the 20th century, many events happened that still influence us now. The first of them was Britain's switch to a nationalized healthcare system in 1948, which required a reevaluation of whether procedures were actually necessary for light of the new cost-benefit analysis. Circumcision rates fell sharply throughout Europe after Gairdner's 1949 article on the natural history of the foreskin [5].

In the early 1970s, the Australian Pediatrics Association and the Canadian Pediatric Society recommended against routine circumcision, and rates subsequently declined in those countries as well. Alanis and Lucidi [10] explained that the rates of circumcision fell only slightly in the United States despite official policy statements by the American Academy of Pediatrics (AAP) Task Force on Circumcision in 1971, 1975, and 1977 that circumcision "offered no medical benefit during the neonatal period". These authors [10] also wrote that in 1989, the AAP modified its position on circumcision after more evidence came to light that it effectively reduced male urinary tract infections and sexually transmitted diseases, and in 1999 the AAP returned to a more negative view on routine circumcision with the following official policy statement: "Existing scientific evidence demonstrates potential medical benefits of newborn male circumcision; however, these data are not sufficient to recommend routine neonatal circumcision". On the other hand, the 2012 AAP statement stated that an assessment of the most recent research indicates that the health benefits of neonatal male circumcision exceed the risks and that the procedure's advantages warrant access to it for families who choose to have it [13]. The reduction of penile cancer, genital herpes, and some sexually transmitted illnesses, such as HIV, were among the specific advantages noted.

3. Circumcision from a ritual or religious perspective

3.1 Judaism

Judaism is a culture that practices circumcision in a ritual religious manner. Several authors [1, 3, 6, 7, 9–12, 14, 15] explain in the following paragraph when religious practice began and how it remains in force until our times. Bris Milah, or Jewish ritual circumcision, is performed on the eighth day of life to fulfill the Covenant between God and Abraham in which God set his seal on Abraham and his descendants (Gén. 17:10–14). Just as Abraham circumcised his son Isaac (Gen. 21:4), so the child's father must ensure that his children bear the mark of this covenant, which distinguishes Israel as God's chosen people (**Figure 2**). Without this symbol of recommitment and cleansing, neither the Paschal celebration (Ex. 12:48), which celebrates Israel's freedom from

DOI: http://dx.doi.org/10.5772/intechopen.106533

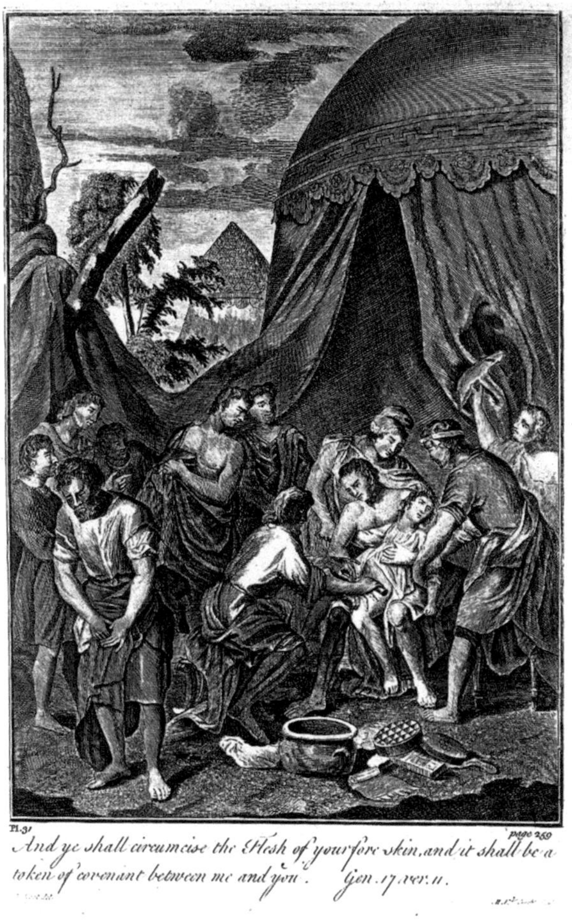

Figure 2.
Abraham and his men begin to circumcise themselves. Etching by M. van der Gucht after G. Hoet. Hoet, Gerard, 1648–1733. Wellcome collection. Public domain mark.

slavery in Egypt nor the making of a covenant with a Jewish family, could be commemorated (Gen 34:14–16). The mohels, or master circumcisers, incorporated specialized tools, the Izmel, a double-edged knife to excise the prepuce, and later, the Mogen shield to protect the glans. Both Orthodox and Reformed Judaism still conduct circumcisions on all males worldwide. While Reform Jews permit a doctor to execute the process, in Orthodox Judaism the rite is carried out by a mohel, an ordained authority. It is thought that God will punish the father by reducing his lifespan if he fails to carry out this duty to have his child circumcised. Exceptions to the circumcision obligation are mentioned in the Talmud, the codification and interpretation of the Torah, recorded by Jewish scholars in the 4th, 5th, and 6th centuries AD. For example, in case of illness, circumcision should be postponed until the boy is better. It is also described in the Talmud that if a woman loses two sons or if two sisters each lose a son because of circumcision, which in most cases is caused by exsanguination, the following sons of her or other sisters within the same family do not need to be circumcised. This is considered the first reference to hemophilia, a condition inherited through the maternal line.

3.2 Christianity

As can be read in the New Testament, Jesus of Nazareth was circumcised (Gospel according to Luke, chapter 2) (**Figure 3**). John the Baptist was also circumcised (chapter 1). Furthermore, Jesus of Nazareth never spoke against circumcision. However, circumcision has not become part of Christian traditions. This is attributed to Paul, who emphasizes in several of his letters that physical circumcision is not a prerequisite for salvation but involves spiritual circumcision of the heart ('Letter to the Romans', chapter 2) [9].

3.3 Islam

Muslims adopted ritual circumcision as well. Usually carried out by older boys as a pubertal transition to adulthood. Although the Koran makes no mention of circumcision, its development can be traced to the Sunnah (the sayings and deeds of the prophet Mohammed) [1, 6, 7, 10]. Other authors [9, 15] are of the opinion that the practice is attributed to the prophet Abraham, whom Muslims, like Jews, revere as patriarch. Muslims are divided into six different schools of thought within Islam and there are differences of opinion between these schools about the rules for circumcision. Among the schools, only the Shafiites consider it obligatory while for the others it is simply recommended. The Prophet Mohammed recommended performing circumcision on the 7th day after birth, but it can be performed up to 7 years [3, 7, 9, 15].

3.4 Other cultures

Two of the oldest still-practicing versions of Christianity are practiced by Coptic Christians in Egypt and Ethiopian Orthodox Christians, who maintain many aspects of early Christianity, such as male circumcision (for example, 97 percent of Orthodox men in Ethiopia are circumcised). While some Christian congregations in South

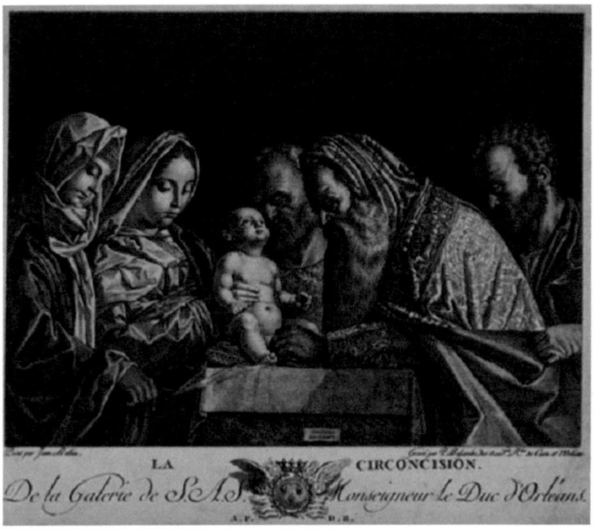

Figure 3.
The circumcision of Christ. Oil painting after Hendrik Goltzius. Goltzius, Hendrik, 1558–1617. Wellcome library no. 44858i. Reproduced with permission of the Wellcome institute.

Africa reject the practice and view it as a sacrificial activity, others, like the Nomiya Church in Kenya, demand circumcision as a condition of membership. In Malawi and Zambia, some groups expressed similar views that Christians should perform circumcision since Jesus underwent the procedure and the Bible endorses it [3 p. 4].

Numerous ethnic groups around the world have all practiced circumcision for non-religious purposes for many centuries, including the Australian Aborigines, the Aztecs, and the Mayans, as well as communities of the Philippines, eastern Indonesia, and several Pacific islands, including Fiji and the Polynesian islands. Although it may have initially been a test of fortitude and endurance, circumcision is now a necessary component of a rite of passage into manhood in the majority of these societies. As boys of the same age are circumcised at the same time, circumcision also contributes to social cohesion, masculinity, self-identity, and spirituality.

4. History of circumcision techniques

4.1 Description of the technique in ancient times

In the Eberst papyrus (Egypt) and later in the Bible (Exodus, chapter 4:25–26 and Joshua, chapter 5:2–8) only reference is made to circumcision being performed with a knife [1, 9].

4.2 Medieval medicine

In the Middle Ages, the circumcision technique was described by the French surgeon Guy de Chauliac (c. 1360). Circumcision is performed by taking the foreskin between the fingertips and pulling it over the glans towards the end of the penis. The foreskin is excised distal to the glans with a scalpel, after which hemostasis is performed with red powder or by cauterization [9].

One of the earliest descriptions of Muslim circumcision is given by the 15th-century Ottoman surgeon Serefeddin Sabuncuoglu. He recommends creating two ligatures, between which the foreskin can be safely cut. During the procedure, the wound is covered with dry pumpkin ash or white flour, and then a bandage is applied [9].

4.3 From the 19th century up today

The first surgical papers detailing circumcision started to appear in medical texts in the mid-19th century. The fundamental surgical principles that are still in use today are fully described by Sir Frederick Treves in his work from 1903 (**Figure 4**) [1, 5]. Like the majority of his colleagues, he used scissors to remove the foreskin (**Figure 5**), and he states that adult patients must have the frenular artery tied. He makes it very clear that you must leave enough inner skin exposed because doing otherwise can lead to synechiae. Treves also asserts that interrupted fine catgut sutures must be used for the skin's appositional sutures [1, 5].

The antihemorrhagic triradiate continuous circumcision suture line was described by the French surgeon E. Doyen and his English co-author H. Spencer-Browne. Three circular sutures made of no. 1 silk, each one-third the circle of the glans, were employed to "coaptate" the borders of the skin. To enable expansion of the area between the two skin layers if necessary, the ends were left untied (**Figure 6**) [1, 5].

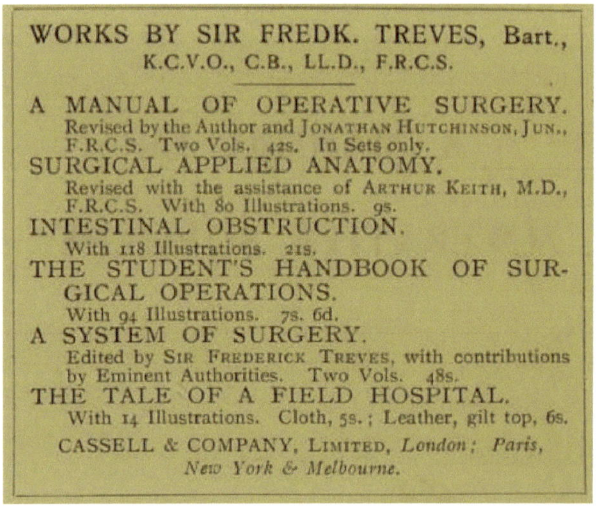
WORKS BY SIR FREDK. TREVES, Bart.,
K.C.V.O., C.B., LL.D., F.R.C.S.

A MANUAL OF OPERATIVE SURGERY.
Revised by the Author and JONATHAN HUTCHINSON, JUN., F.R.C.S. Two Vols. 42s. In Sets only.
SURGICAL APPLIED ANATOMY.
Revised with the assistance of ARTHUR KEITH, M.D., F.R.C.S. With 80 Illustrations. 9s.
INTESTINAL OBSTRUCTION.
With 118 Illustrations. 21s.
THE STUDENT'S HANDBOOK OF SURGICAL OPERATIONS.
With 94 Illustrations. 7s. 6d.
A SYSTEM OF SURGERY.
Edited by SIR FREDERICK TREVES, with contributions by Eminent Authorities. Two Vols. 48s.
THE TALE OF A FIELD HOSPITAL.
With 14 Illustrations. Cloth, 5s.; Leather, gilt top, 6s.
CASSELL & COMPANY, LIMITED, *London; Paris, New York & Melbourne.*

Figure 4.
A manual of operative surgery/by sir Frederick Treves. Treves, Frederick, 1853–1923. Date 1903. Volume 190,301. Reproduced with permission of the Wellcome collection. Attribution-noncommercial 4.0 international (CC BY-NC 4.0).

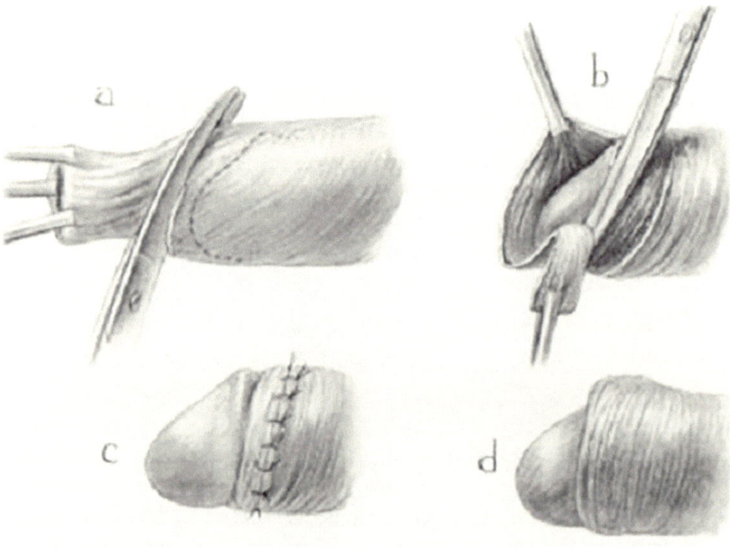

Figure 5.
The scissor technique was described by sir Frederick Treves (1903).

These modifications in suture application are meant to reduce hemorrhage, which is the most common acute consequence. In fact, Charles Chetwood's well-known urological text from 1921 advised leaving long, interrupted horse-hair sutures in place (**Figure** 7). Up to Sir Alec Badenoch's Manual of Urology in 1953 [5], variations of what came to be known as "Chetwood's dressing" were documented.

At the beginning of the 20th century, techniques for circumcision in neonates began to be described. Carrying out the procedure in the neonatal period, it was shown that the manual compression of the surgical bed was able to control the

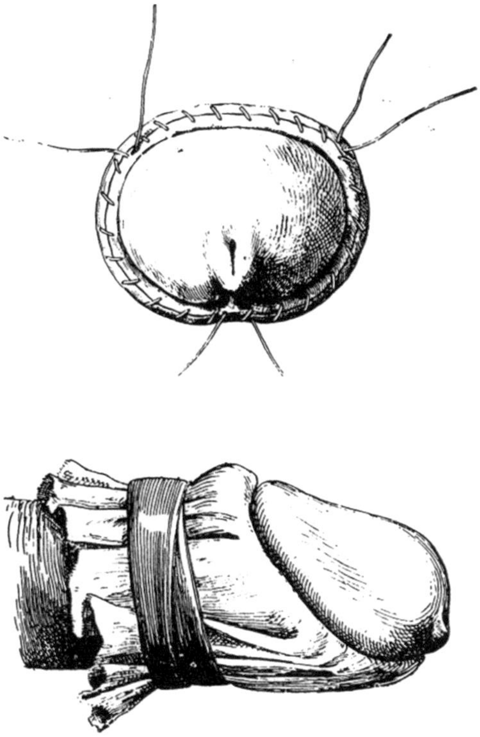

Figure 6.
The triradiate continuous suture of doyen (1920) and compressive muslin dressing.

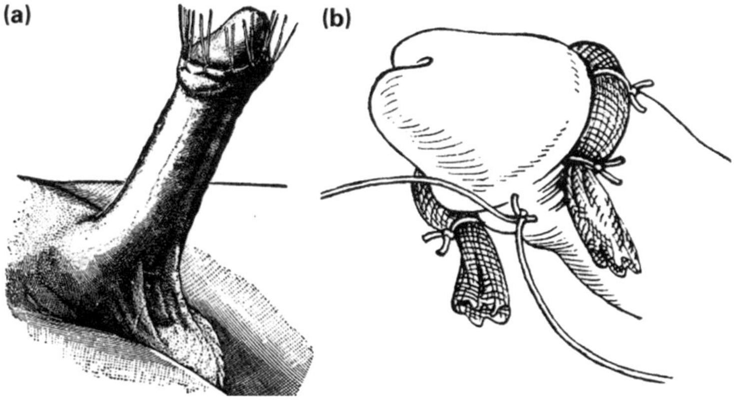

Figure 7.
(a) Chetwood's long horse-hair tethering sutures (1921) and (b) Chetwood's dressing.

hemorrhage. Subsequently, with this acquired knowledge, instruments were created for hemostatic purposes to perform surgery in this group of patients [1]. The first device was Doyen's E'craseur (1920). The foreskin was compressed and then cut by this instrument, which controlled bleeding after surgery without the need to use a hemostatic suture. This technique is also used in adults (**Figure 8**) [1, 5].

Many circumcision clamps were available for use on neonates by the 1930s. The Winkelman prototype was first presented in 1935, and as of this writing, it still

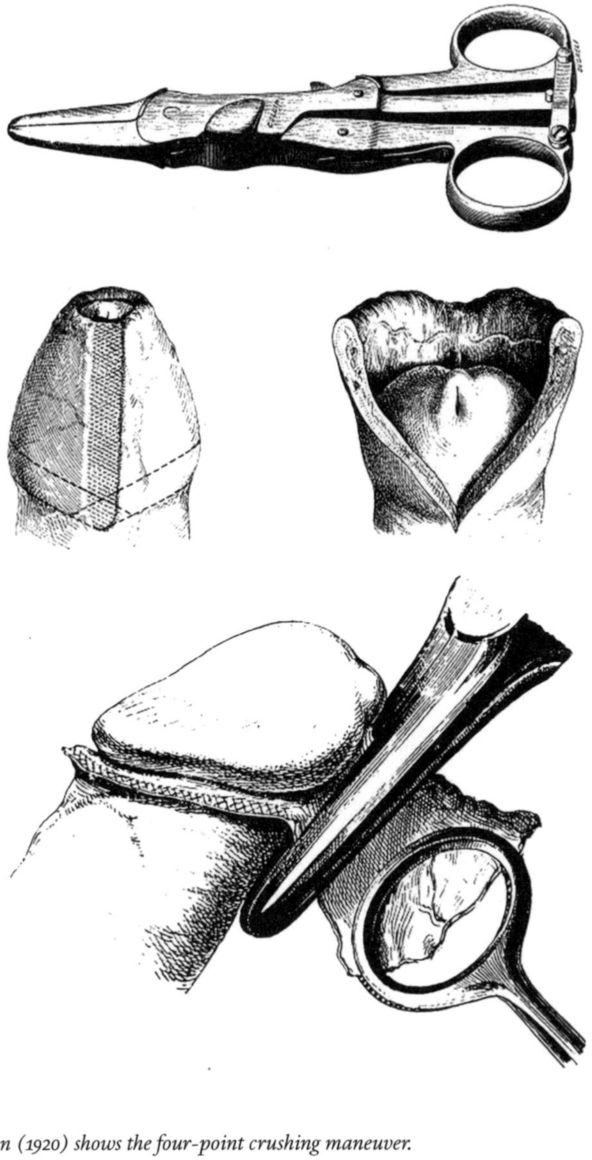

Figure 8.
The E'craseur of doyen (1920) shows the four-point crushing maneuver.

maintains a mostly unchanged appearance (**Figure 9**) [1, 5]. In 1940 another circumcision device was introduced (**Figure 10**) [1]. The Gomco clamp offers excellent esthetic results with little to no bleeding, shorter surgical times, and a short learning curve. It is, however, only applicable during the newborn period [1, 16]. The device featured a bell and a base plate. The Gomco bell was placed over the glans at the level of the crown and the foreskin was brought back into the anatomical position. A tensioning bar that looped under a T-shaped part at the top of the bell and was fastened to the metal plate kept the foreskin in place. After the foreskin had been sufficiently strangled, the prepuce was cut using a scalpel [17, 18].

In 1939, Dr. Cecil J. Ross patented steel circumcision rings, and from this invention came the idea of using a tourniquet method for circumcision [18]. The "Plastibell gadget" was developed in the 1950s (**Figure 11**). In 1956 it began to be used for neonates

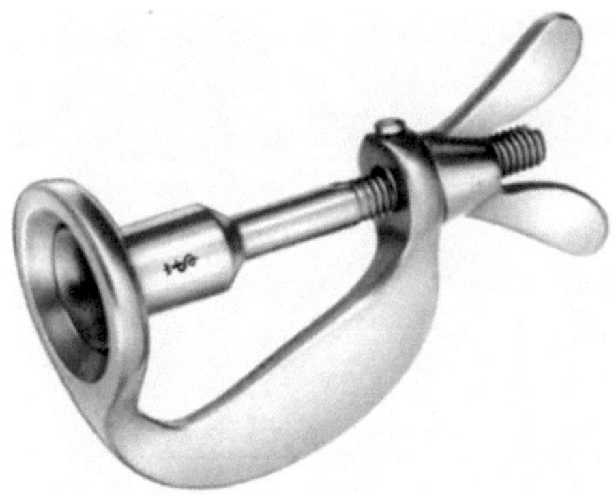

Figure 9.
The 'Winkelman' circumcision clamp. Reproduced with permission of Aescalup surgical products.

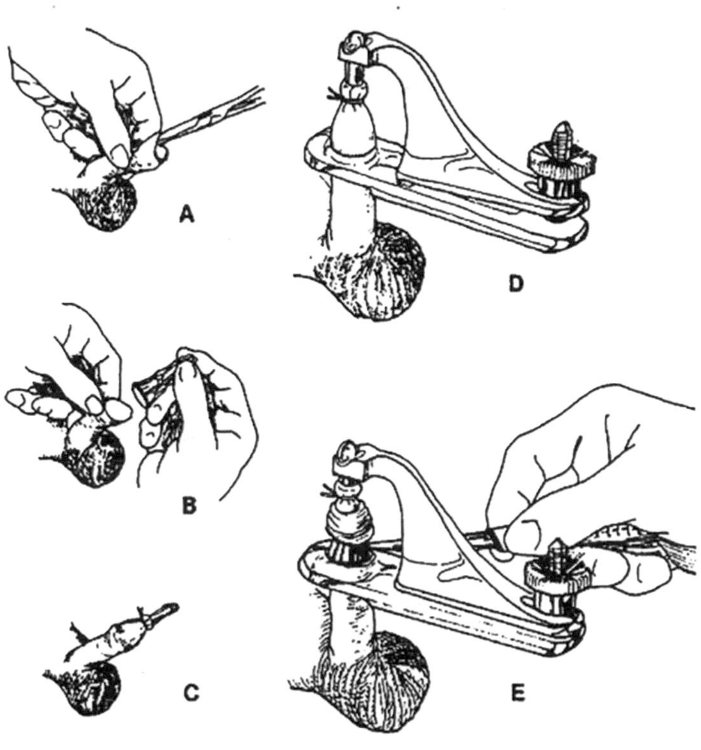

Figure 10.
The Gomco technique.

and later its use was extended to the present for all pediatric patients [1, 5, 9, 16]. A plastic bell is placed covering the glans and then the foreskin covers the bell and a ligature is made around the foreskin. Placing the ligature around the foreskin breaks the handle of the cup, which is left open until it falls off, which happens in about 7 to 10 days [17, 18].

Dr. Harry Bronstein introduced The Mogen clamp as a different tool in 1955 (**Figure 12**) [16]. This clamp has a small slit through which the foreskin is placed once it is slid and separated from the glans, and then pulled with a hemostatic

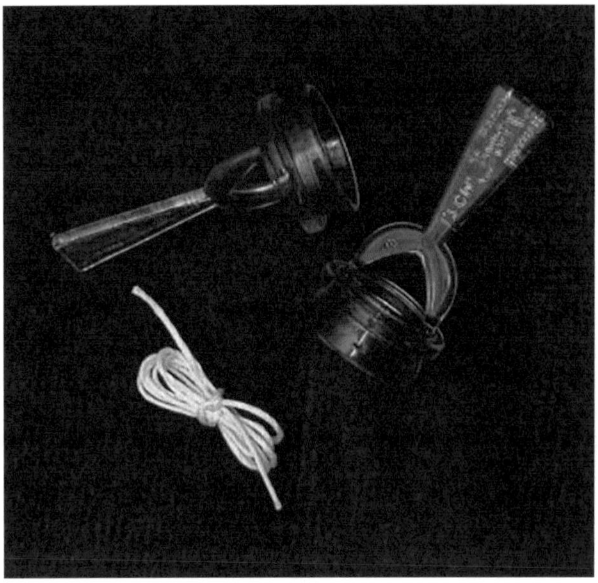

Figure 11.
The Plastibell device.

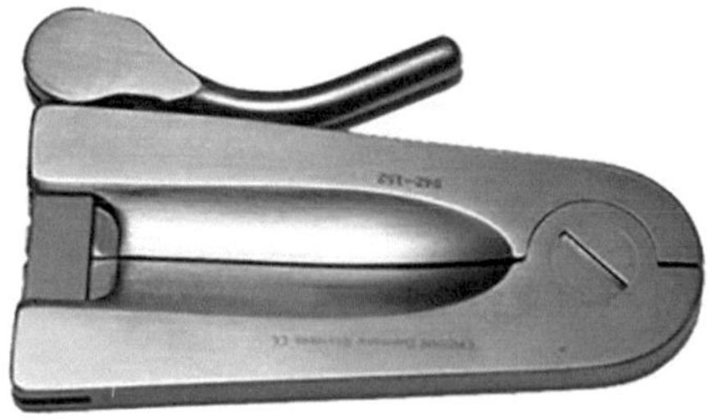

Figure 12.
The Mogen clamp.

clamp. After placement, it is cut with the scalpel, when there is the confidence that the glans is not included. The incision is simply wrapped to establish hemostasis; no stitches are used [17, 18].

In 2003 a new circumcision device was invented. The device made in China was called the Shang Ring by its creator J. Shang (**Figure 13**). This device facilitated its widespread use due to its easy applicability and was incorporated in several countries with the aim of preventing HIV infection, for which the World Health Organization approved its use. It presents a short learning curve for health personnel who incorporate it into their practice [17, 18]. The device features two rings, one internal and one external. The inner ring is placed in the coronal sulcus, and the foreskin is placed over the inner ring. The outer ring is then placed and the excess foreskin is removed with scissors. In 7 days the hemostatic ring can be removed. This technique does not use sutures [17, 18].

Another device manufactured for use in adults on a large scale was the PrePex device. It was patented in 2011 and the objective of its creation was also to apply it massively in HIV prevention programs. The device has a ring that is inserted into the

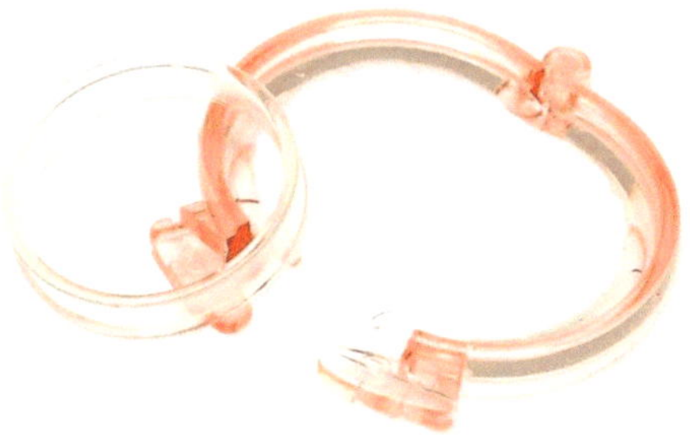

Figure 13.
The Shang ring device.

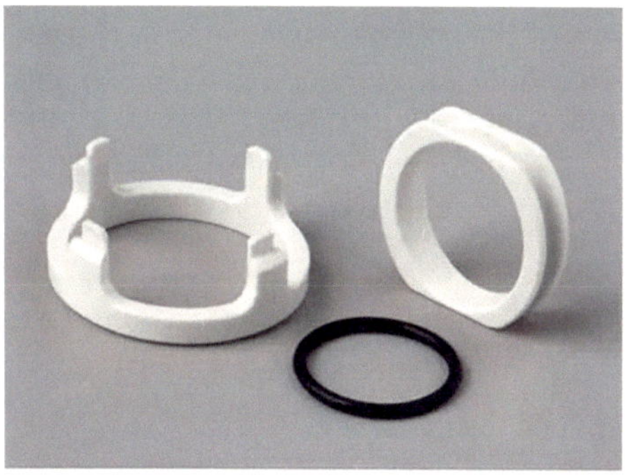

Figure 14.
The PrePex device.

foreskin on the glans and another elastic outer ring. The compression generated by these two rings generates necrosis and subsequent fall of the foreskin approximately 7 days after placement (**Figure 14**) [17, 18].

There are other devices created for circumcision that have been validated but have not gained as much popularity as those described above. One interesting is the "Circumplast" is one of them used in neonates and pediatric patients and consists of a plastic bell provided with a handle with its ligature. A characteristic of the instruments is that allow the physician to see the glans. Additionally visible through the skin is the Circumplast's proximal lip, which serves as a visual cue to confirm the device's correct positioning. If the ligature is positioned improperly or if there is too much internal mucous membrane, the surgeon can change its position [19].

5. Conclusion

Circumcision, a procedure at least 5000 years old, with profound religious and cultural significance, will predictably continue as a feature of human living for many generations to come.

More research is necessary to determine which culture first initiated the circumcision practice, so we think that all of the theories mentioned are probably partially correct.

It has been done for many reasons from religious, passage of rituals, traditional and hygienic reasons and for prevention of diseases ranging from sexually transmitted diseases. Independientemente del motivo de su realización hoy en día es una práctica frecuente tanto como causas religiosas, médicas o rituales.

For medical causes in which circumcision is indicated, there has been a major technological advance since the first description of the technique in medical books. These advances try to facilitate the use of devices that can be used by medical and non-medical personnel for the prevention of sexually transmitted diseases in places where the incidence of them is worrying.

Despite all, circumcision seems to permeate all of humanity from early ancient times to the technologically developed modern world.

Acknowledgements

This report is the result of the collaborative work of the teaching and research team at Hospital San Bernardo in the province of Salta, Argentina. The report was written by Claudio Militello and Veronica Pais.

Conflict of interest

"The authors declare no conflict of interest."

Author details

Claudio Militello* and Veronica Pais
San Bernardo Hospital, Salta, Argentina

*Address all correspondence to: c_militello_bellomo@hotmail.com

References

[1] Totaro A, Volpe A, Racioppi M, Pinto F, Sacco E, Bassi PF. Circumcision: History, religion and law. Urologia Journal. 2011;**78**(1):1-9. DOI: 10.5301/RU.2011.6433

[2] Falcão B, Stegani M, Matias J. Phimosis and circumcision: Concepts, history, and evolution. International Journal of Medical Reviews. 2018;**5**(1): 6-18. DOI: 10.29252/IJMR-050103World Health

[3] World Health Organization. Male Circumcision: Global Trends and Determinants of Prevalence, Safety and Acceptability. No. UNAIDS/07.29 E/JC1320E. Geneva (CH): World Health Organization; 2008. p. 30

[4] Morris BJ, Wamai RG, Henebeng EB, Tobian AA, Klausner JD, Banerjee J, et al. Estimation of country-specific and global prevalence of male circumcision. Population Health Metrics. 2016;**14**(1): 1-13. DOI: 10.1186/s12963-016-0073-5

[5] Dunsmuir WD, Gordon EM. The history of circumcision. BJU International. 1999;**83**(S1):1-12. DOI: 10.1046/j.1464-410x.1999.0830s1001.x

[6] Doyle D. Ritual male circumcision: A brief history. The Journal of the Royal College of Physicians of Edinburgh. 2005;**35**(3):279-285

[7] Prabhakaran S, Ljuhar D, Coleman R, Nataraja RM. Circumcision in the pediatric patient: A review of indications, technique, and complications. Journal of Paediatrics and Child Health. 2018;**54**(12):1299-1307. DOI: 10.1111/jpc.14206

[8] Brondz I, Aslanova T. Circumcision: History, scope, and aim: Part I. Voice of the Publisher. 2019;**5**:77-87. DOI: 10.4236/vp.2019.54006

[9] Meijer B, Butzelaar RM. Circumcisie in historisch perspectief. Nederlands tijdschrift voor geneeskunde. 2000;**144**(52):2504-2508

[10] Alanis MC, Lucidi RS. Neonatal circumcision: A review of the world's oldest and most controversial operation. Obstetrical & Gynecological Survey. 2004;**59**(5):379-395. DOI: 10.1097/00006254-200405000-00026

[11] Allan N. Illustrations from the Wellcome institute library. A polish rabbi's circumcision manual. Medical History. 1989;**33**(2):247-254. DOI: 10.1017/s0025727300049279

[12] Raveenthiran V. The evolutionary saga of circumcision from a religious perspective. Journal of Pediatric Surgery. 2018;**53**(7):1440-1443. DOI: 10.1016/j.jpedsurg.2018.03.001

[13] Blank S, Brady M, Buerk E, Carlo W, Diekema D, Freedman A, et al. American Academy of Pediatrics task force on circumcision. Circumcision policy statement. Pediatrics. 2012;*130*(3): 585-586. DOI: 10.1542/peds.2012-1989

[14] El-Gohary MA. Circumcision: History, philosophy and facts. Open Journal of Urology. 2015;**5**(08):114

[15] Zampieri N, Pianezzola E, Zampieri C. Male circumcision through the ages: The role of tradition. Acta Paediatrica. 2008;**97**(9):1305-1307. DOI: 10.1111/j.1651-2227.2008.00917.x

[16] Krill AJ, Palmer LS, Palmer JS. Complications of circumcision.

The Scientific World Journal. 2011;**11**: 2458-2468. DOI: 10.1100/2011/373829

[17] Abdulwahab-Ahmed A, Mungadi IA. Techniques of male circumcision. Journal of Surgical Technique and Case Report. 2013;**5**(1): 1-7. DOI: 10.4103/2006-8808.118588

[18] World Health Organization, JHPIEGO. Manual for early infant male circumcision under local anaesthesia. Geneva (CH): World Health Organization; 2010. p. 127

[19] World Health Organization. WHO technical advisory group on innovations in male circumcision, meeting report; 30 September - 2 October 2014, Geneva, Switzerland. Geneva (CH): World Health Organization; 2015. pp. 2-35

Chapter 3

Circumcision Clamps for Adults

Cristina M. Fernández-Ávila, Rodrigo García-Baquero and José Luis Álvarez-Ossorio

Abstract

Circumcision is one of the surgical interventions with the longest historical tradition for various medical or non-medical, religious and social, reasons. Due to a high demand for this surgery, in recent years, a large number of plastic and disposable devices have emerged in order to optimize the technique. Although they were initially used in newborns and children, their use in recent years has been expanding to adults. The main objectives of these devices are to shorten the surgical time, simplify the technique, and maintain an adequate safety profile compared to the classic suture technique. All reviewed devices for adult circumcision appear to achieve these goals, making them a safe, fast, and feasible option for use in an outpatient setting or in high-demand areas.

Keywords: circumcision, plastic rings, adults, foreskin, phimosis

1. Introduction

Circumcision is one of the surgical interventions with the longest historical tradition for religious, mainly Muslim and Jewish, social and medical reasons with the aim of promoting hygiene and reducing the incidence of sexually transmitted diseases (HIV, human papilloma virus, and the herpes simplex virus) [1]. Many observational studies and three large randomized controlled trials conducted in Kenya, Uganda, and Orange Farm, South Africa, show that male circumcision reduces female-to-male HIV transmission by 60% [2] and even prevents penile cancer (Africa and South America). The World Health Organization (WHO) in 2007 recommended this surgery with the aim of reducing the incidence rates of sexually transmitted diseases in countries with high prevalence.

In developed countries, the surgical indication is usually purely medical, with phimosis being the main indication. There are also other pathologies that benefit from this intervention such as paraphimosis, balanitis (inflammation of the foreskin), posthitis (inflammation of the glans), localized condyloma acuminata, and localized carcinomas. For all these reasons, the demand is high and constant.

Around 25–33% of the world's total male population is circumcised [3], but this rate varies widely depending on the country analyzed. In the US, an average of one million newborn boys are circumcised annually. The circumcision rate in the US is as high as 70%, while in Britain it is 6%. In Nigeria, the circumcision rate is estimated at 87% [4]. Despite being such a frequent surgery, it is not exempt from complications, although the incidence is low when adequate sanitary conditions are met (2–4%) [5].

There are currently several surgical techniques to perform circumcision, but in general they can be classified into two large groups depending on the material used to adhere the cut edges and maintain hemostasis, regardless of the foreskin excision technique. In conventional circumcision, the cut edges of the wound are held together with sutures. The alternative technique known as minimally invasive circumcision uses a plastic device. These approximate the wound edges and control hemostasis. The goals of these devices are to achieve a safer, easier, and faster procedure, faster healing than conventional methods, require less surgical experience, and generate better esthetic results. Each surgical technique has its own limitations and risk–benefit ratios.

2. Classic technique with suture

Circumcision surgery is such a widespread surgery that, depending on the surgeon who performs it, it may undergo different modifications, but it must always comply with some basic premises: adequate asepsis and hemostasis, excision of the outer and inner preputial skin layers and protection of the glans and urethra during the procedure in order to avoid complications. We must also seek a satisfactory esthetic result for the patient.

In general, this technique consists of a dorsal incision until the glans can be uncovered and a subsequent circumferential incision approximately 1 cm from the balanopreputial sulcus. In the ventral part, the frenulum is sectioned, leaving the circumferential incision in the form of an inverted "V" at that level. This incision should traverse the dartos to reach Buck's fascia. Next, we must suture the frenulum longitudinally with two to four points with 4/0 absorbable suture. With the foreskin reduced (not covering the glans), a second circumferential incision is made following the relief of the balanopreputial groove. Finally, we must excise the sleeve of skin that remains between the two incisions made, coagulate all the bleeding vessels and suture the edges of the wound with the same suture used previously. To carry out this suture, it is advisable to first make some cardinal points of reference and then give a few loose stiches between the initially given reference stiches. All this is carried out under local anesthesia. It requires 4 to 6 weeks of abstinence from sexual activity to allow complete wound healing.

Open surgical techniques require surgical experience and at least 20 minutes of operative time. They have a high rate of minor complications (mainly hematoma, bleeding, infection, and delayed healing), which decrease with surgical experience [6].

3. Disponsable devices for adult circumcision

Recently, a series of minimally invasive techniques performed with plastic devices have emerged. This type of sutureless device has traditionally been more studied and used in children. We will focus our review on the devices currently available in adults and their possible advantages.

These types of devices generally sandwich the mucous and cutaneous layer of the foreskin between two concentric rings, one inside and one outside. The glans is usually protected by placing a bell-shaped protector between the two on the glans. These devices act in the form of a clamp, cutting off the blood supply to the distal part of the foreskin. This can be excised or left to necrotize. Most of these devices must be kept in place for a week before removal, which allows circumcision without sutures. The procedure is ideal for outpatient settings or for use by healthcare personnel with basic surgical knowledge.

However, the beginning of the concept of disposable devices arose with the introduction of metallic instruments to facilitate the surgical incision during circumcision. Although these devices are made of reusable metal, we wanted to add them to this chapter as it is one of the pioneering techniques in sutureless circumcision surgery. They are the Gomco and the Mogen clamps.

Gomco clamp

The Gomco clamp was launched in 1935 in the US. It has traditionally been used in neonates, especially in the US, but its use has been expanded to adults. The main difference between both groups is that in adulthood we need to suture the edges of the wound in order to avoid bleeding, specially once the patient begins to move and notice erections, obviously stronger to that of neonates or children. However, this issue was questioned when studies in 2002 demonstrated the superiority of tissue adhesives over suture closure in circumcisions [7, 8]. These reduce operative time, improve cosmetic outcome, and increase patient satisfaction [8].

Removal of the foreskin with the Gomco forceps and sealing of the wound edges with tissue adhesive results in a minimally invasive circumcision that is easy to perform, heals quickly, and has excellent cosmetic results [9]. In a study by Millard et al., this device was compared with the classic suture technique in adults. The authors concluded that the Gomco device with the tissue adhesive required much less operative time, was easier to perform, had much better cosmetic results, and was potentially safer than open surgery. It takes 1–2 min to place the Gomco instrument, 5 min to wait, and 2–3 min to remove and apply the adhesive (**Figure 1**) [9].

Mogen clamp.

By this instrument, the foreskin is stretched distal to the glans and a metal shield is slipped over the foreskin just distal to the glans. A scalpel is used to remove the redundant distal foreskin. The frenulum is not involved in the excision. The Mogen clamp is held for a few minutes, and a bandage is then placed to prevent bleeding (**Figure 2**).

Moving back to the disposable devices, there are a large number of them of which we will just analyze the most used today (**Table 1**).

3.1 Alisklamp

This clamp system is supplied in two parts, a clear polycarbonate tube and a white plastic clamping mechanism. He achieves circumcision by crushing the foreskin

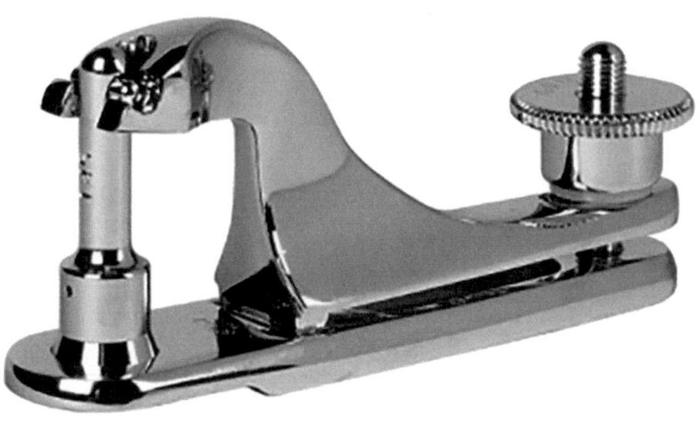

Figure 1.
Gomco clamp device [10].

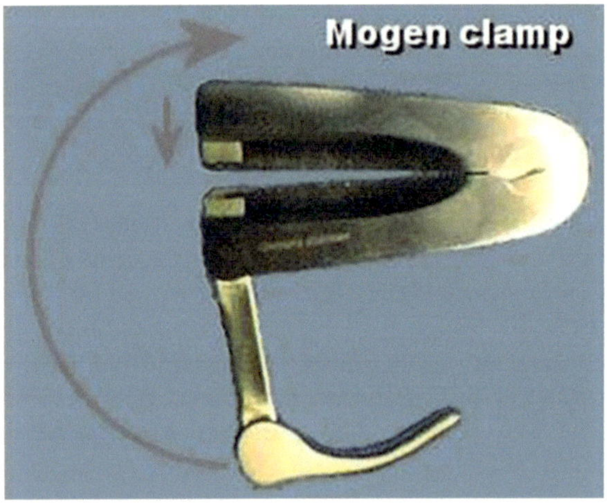

Figure 2.
Mogen clamp device [11].

Male circumcision devices
Accucirc ® (Safecirc clinic, Wakefeld, United State)
AlisKlamp ® (Healing Hands Clinic, Ankara)
Circumplast ® (Emboss Medical Limited, United Kingdom)
Ismail clamp ® (Drims Trading Sdn Bhd, Malaysia)
Plastibell ® (Advin Health Care, India)
PrePex ® (Circ MedTech, Hod Hasharon, Israel)
ShangRing ® (Wuhu Snnda Medical Treatment Appliance Technology, China)
SmartClamp ® (GoDaddy Operating Company, United State)
SurgiPex ® (Dynamic experts, Pakistán)
Tara Klamp ® (Tara Medic Corporation Sdn. Bhd, Malaysia)
Unicirc ® (Unicirc Pty Ltd., South Africa)
Winkelmann clamp
Zhenxi rings ® (Weihai Zhenxi Medical Equipment Corporation, South Korean)

Table 1.
List of currently available male circumcision devices.

between the two components. Excess tissue is removed with a scalpel, but that cut does not define the scar line; scalpel cutting simply removes what would otherwise become a mass of necrotic tissue. The most frequent complications were excessive foreskin (0.7%), followed by bleeding (0.6%), infection (0.55%), wound dehiscence (0.25%), buried penis (0.25%), and urine retention (0.1%) (**Figure 3**) [11].

3.2 Plastibell

A plastic bell with a slit in the proximal part is slipped between the glans and the foreskin, and suture material is tied tightly. The suture produces necrosis, with the distal foreskin falling off in 7–10 days (**Figure 4**).

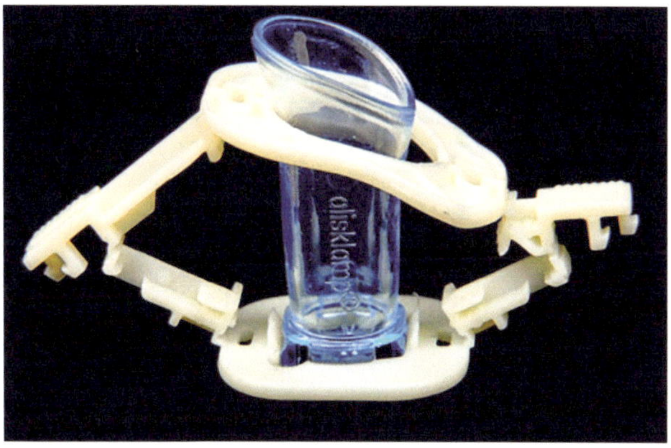

Figure 3.
Alisklamp device [12].

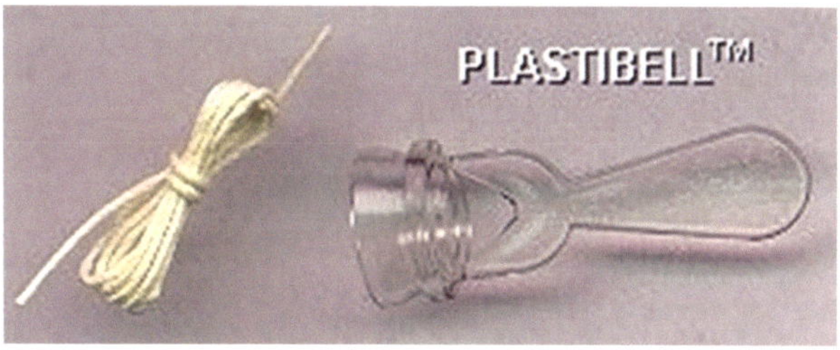

Figure 4.
Plastibell device [11].

3.3 Prepex

It consists of an inner ring, an elastic ring, a locating ring, and a verification thread. It has been approved by the US Food and Drug Administration (FDA) and carries a European mark of conformity (EC). To place the device, we must place the elastic ring on the placement ring. The placement ring is then left at the base of the penis, and the inner ring is inserted between the glans and the foreskin. The elastic ring is deployed between the placement and the inner rings at the circumcision line. This compresses the foreskin and cuts off distal circulation, causing necrosis and allowing it to be excised within 7 days after device placement without bleeding. The Prepex device can be applied and removed without the need for local anesthesia and has potential for use in non-sterile settings with limited resources (**Figure 5**) [14].

3.4 Shang ring

It is the most studied device, easy and fast to apply under local anesthesia. It is one of the devices prequalified by the WHO for use in adolescent and adult circumcision. It has also received FDA approval for use in adults, in addition to EC mark [15]. The estimated surgical time in adults is 3 to 5 minutes [16, 17]. The circumference of the penis must be measured accurately, and it is important to calculate the correct size. The device is available in 32 sizes to fit all ages, from newborns to adults. It is safe and effective in both adolescents and adults, with a success rate of the procedure greater than 99%. No serious adverse effects were reported (**Figure 6**) [19].

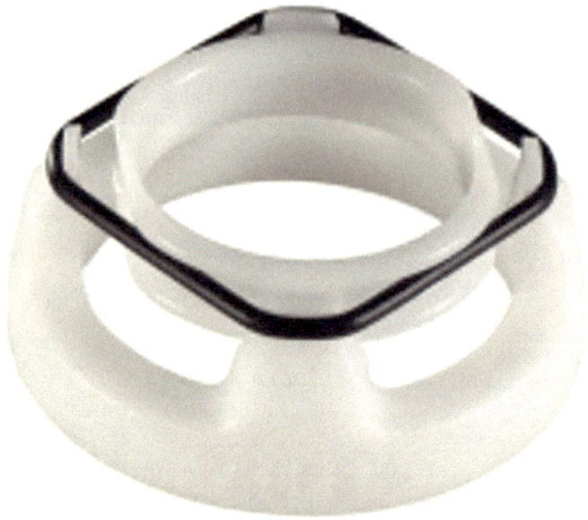

Figure 5.
Prepex device [13].

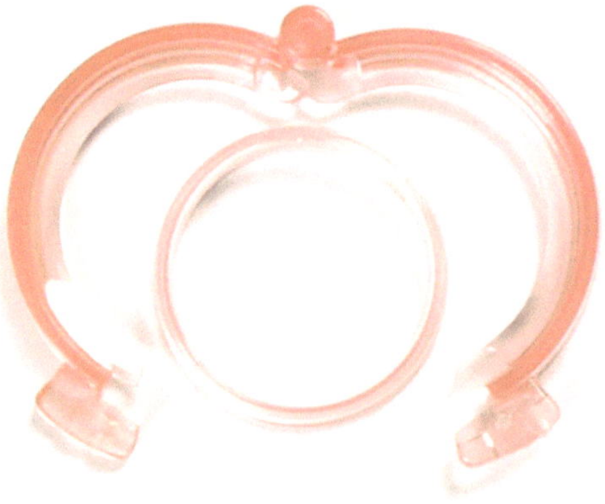

Figure 6.
Shang ring device [18].

3.5 Unicirc

It works very similar to the Gomco clamp. After the application of the device on the glans, the foreskin is placed on the transparent bell and adjusted accordingly. The device is then screwed on tightly and held in place for 5 minutes, bringing the mucosal and skin surfaces together to minimize bleeding while the foreskin is removed. The Unicirc is then removed and a cyanoacrylate adhesive is applied to promote healing by primary intention. The first version of the device resulted in higher postoperative blood loss compared to open surgery, prompting a change in the setting of the mechanism to ensure adequate hemostasis (**Figure** 7) [9].

The literature seems to support the results of these devices in terms of efficacy and safety. Hohlfeld et al. state in their review published in Cochrane that the operative time is probably about 17 minutes shorter when a device is used instead of standard

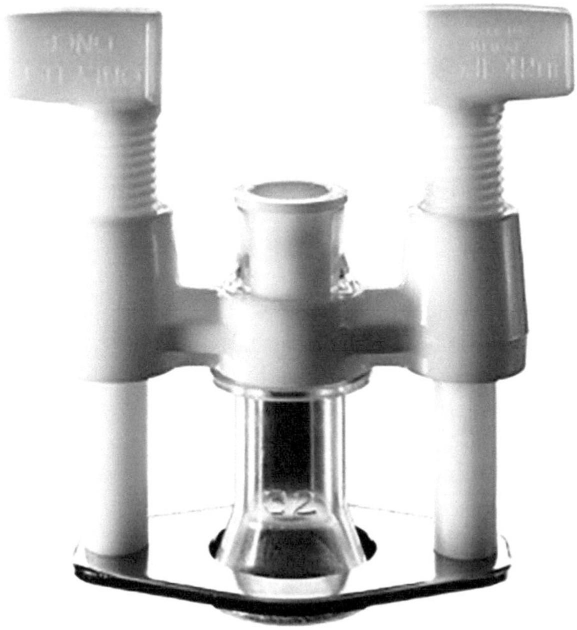

Figure 7.
Unicirc device [20].

surgical techniques, which constitutes a clinically significant decrease in the procedure [21]. The suture surgical technique generally takes about 24 minutes. Another of the items studied in this review was pain. Hohlfeld et al. conclude that there is less postoperative pain during the first 24 hours when circumcision devices are used compared to standard surgical techniques (measured by visual analog scale (VAS)). Beyond those first few hours, there is little or no difference in postoperative pain experienced up to the first 7 days compared with standard surgical techniques [21]. In terms of adverse effects, when a circumcision device is used compared to a standard surgical technique, there are probably no more serious adverse events, such as hospitalization or permanent damage, although there may be a slight increase in moderate adverse events requiring minimal interventions, such as suture or antibiotics. No serious adverse events were reported when circumcision devices were used compared to standard surgical techniques [21, 22].

4. Complications

Weiss et al. reported in a meta-analysis a median frequency of 1.5% (range 0–16%) for any complication from circumcision [23]. The risks and severity of complications are greater with traditional non-medical circumcision than with medical circumcision.

Bleeding. In the suture technique, between 0.1% and 35% have been reported, although transfusion is unusual [24, 25], but if we focus on the device technique, we will discover that the bleeding rates are not usually exceed 1%. Of all the devices, it is especially common in sutureless devices that only use the bandage to control hemostasis (Mogen). In systems such as Gomco or Plastibell, 1% of bleeding has been reported that required some action by the doctor to control it [26].

Glans necrosis. Distal ischemia resulting in such tissue loss may be due to infection, [27] the use of epinephrine-containing local anesthetic agents, attempts at cautery and suture hemostasis, and injudicious and prolonged use of a tourniquet or tight bandage [28]. It is especially common with the use of diathermy with metal clamps (Gomco). Necrosis as a complication of circumcision is very rare [27].

Lack of redundant foreskin droop. It may be due to a poor choice of size or a poor coupling of the device.

Infection. The incidence of infection in a series of neonatal circumcisions was 0.4%, while in a series of older boys it was as high as 10% [11]. Most infections are minor and of little or no importance. Gee et al. notes that infections were significantly more frequent with the Plastibell device than Gomco, even though it has a lower rate of dehiscence or results in removal of too much skin [26].

Urinary retention. This has been reported, after circumcision, secondary to a tight circular bandage [4]. It really is a very rare thing.

Fistula. Most cases have occurred after the use of a clamp-type device where hemostatic sutures were placed on the frenulum with inadvertent suturing of the underlying urethral tissue.

Suture dehiscence. This type of complication is especially mentioned in the works that refer to the Gomco device, where tissue adhesive is used. Although dehiscence rates are low (0–6.8%) [9], especially in children, the use of this material in adults seems to have a higher rate due to the tension that erections can exert on the suture. Despite this, this type of dehiscence usually does not require surgical repair.

5. Satisfaction in the sexual sphere

Since we are evaluating this minimally invasive circumcision technique in adults, we must mention the possible influence of these devices in the sexual sphere. Most of these devices recommend sexual abstinence for the first 4 weeks after surgery. After this time, erectile function and sexual libido in adolescents and adults were not affected by circumcision, and a high satisfaction rate was obtained [29].

6. Conclusions

There is an important variety of devices on the market, but they all seem to be based on the same mechanism, necrosis of the distal foreskin through vascular clamping of excess skin. The procedure is ideal for outpatient settings, where a large number of circumcisions are performed by personnel with less surgical experience.

The male circumcision technique in adults with plastic devices has great advantages over the classic suture technique. The procedure has low complication rates and results in a significant shortening of surgical time. Patients appear to be satisfied with the cosmetic result and experience less pain in the first 24 hours.

Comparative studies between the different devices are currently required in order to elucidate whether any of them stand out from the others in terms of safety and ease of use.

Conflict of interest

The authors declare no conflict of interest.

Appendices and nomenclature

FDA	US Food and Drug Administration
EC	European conformity
WHO	World Health Organization
VAS	visual analog scale

Author details

Cristina M. Fernández-Ávila*, Rodrigo García-Baquero and José Luis Álvarez-Ossorio
Andrology and Reconstructive Urogenital Surgery Unit, Urology Department, Hospital Universitario Puerta del Mar, Cádiz, Spain

*Address all correspondence to: crisferavi@gmail.com

References

[1] Bailey RC, Moses S, Parker CB, Agot K, Maclean I, Krieger JN, et al. Male circumcision for HIV prevention in young men in Kisumu, Kenya: A randomised controlled trial. Lancet. 2007;**369**(9562):643-656. DOI: 10.1016/S0140-6736(07)60312-2

[2] Hargreaves S. 60% reduction in HIV risk with male circumcision, says WHO. The Lancet Infectious Diseases. 2007;7(5):313. DOI: 10.1016/s1473-3099(07)70101-9

[3] Weiss HA. Male circumcision as a preventive measure against HIV and other sexually transmitted diseases. Current Opinion in Infectious Diseases. Feb 2007;**20**(1):66-72

[4] Gerharz EW, Haarmann C. The first cut is the deepest? Medicolegal aspects of male circumcision. BJU International. 2000;**86**(3):332-338. DOI: 10.1046/j.1464-410x.2000.00103.x

[5] Krieger JN, Bailey RC, Opeya JC, Ayieko BO, Opiyo FA, Omondi D, et al. Adult male circumcision outcomes: Experience in a developing country setting. Urologia Internationalis. 2007;**78**(3):235-240. DOI: 10.1159/000099344

[6] Kigozi G, Gray RH, Wawer MJ, Serwadda D, Makumbi F, Watya S, et al. The safety of adult male circumcision in HIV-infected and uninfected men in Rakai, Uganda. PLoS Medicine. 2008;**5**(6):e116. DOI: 10.1371/journal.pmed.0050116

[7] D'Arcy FT, Jaffry SQ. A review of 100 consecutive sutureless child and adult circumcisions. Irish Journal of Medical Science. 2011;**180**(1):51-53. DOI: 10.1007/s11845-010-0545-8

[8] Lane V, Vajda P, Subramaniam R. Paediatric sutureless circumcision: A systematic literature review. Pediatric Surgery International. 2010;**26**(2): 141-144. DOI: 10.1007/s00383-009-2475-y

[9] Millard PS, Wilson HR, Veldkamp PJ, Sitoe N. Rapid, minimally invasive adult voluntary male circumcision: A randomised trial. South African Medical Journal. 2013;**103**(10):736-742. DOI: 10.7196/samj.6856

[10] Gomco clamp device [Internet]. Available from: https://www.alimed.com/gomco-circumcision-clamp.html

[11] Abdulwahab-Ahmed A, Mungadi IA. Techniques of male circumcision. Journal of Surgical Technique and Case Report. 2013;**5**(1): 1-7. DOI: 10.4103/2006-8808.118588

[12] Alisklamp [Internet]. Available from: https://www.facebook.com/alisklampasia/photos/a.335723716774345/335724053440978/

[13] Prepex device [Internet]. Available from: https://finder.startupnationcentral.org/company_page/circ-medtech-prepex#lg=1&slide=2

[14] Bitega JPNM, Hategekimana T, Asiimwe A, Binagwaho A. Safety and Efficacy Study of the PrePex System for Male Circumcision. Boston, USA: Conference on Retroviruses and Opportunistic Infections (CROI); 2011

[15] Al Hussein Alawamlh O, Kim SJ, Li PS, Lee RK. Novel devices for adolescent and adult male circumcision. European Urology Focus. 2018;**4**(3):329-332. DOI: 10.1016/j.euf.2018.06.015

[16] Peng Y, Masson P, Li PS, Chang Y, Tian L, Lee R, et al. No-needle local anesthesia for adult male circumcision. The Journal of Urology. 2010;**184**(3): 978-983. DOI: 10.1016/j.juro.2010.04.080

[17] Senel FM, Demirelli M, Oztek S. Minimally invasive circumcision with a novel plastic clamp technique: A review of 7,500 cases. Pediatric Surgery International. 2010;**26**(7):739-745. DOI: 10.1007/s00383-010-2632-3

[18] Shang Ring device [Internet]. Available from: https://www.researchgate.net/figure/The-Shang-Ring-device_fig 9_221915558

[19] World Health Organization. WHO Technical Advisory Group on Innovations in Male Circumcision: Evaluation of Two Adult Devices, Meeting Report. Geneva, Switzerland: WHO; 2013

[20] Unicirc device [Internet]. Available from: https://unicircglobal.com

[21] Hohlfeld A, Ebrahim S, Shaik MZ, Kredo T. Circumcision devices versus standard surgical techniques in adolescent and adult male circumcisions. Cochrane Database of Systematic Reviews. 2021;**3**(3):CD012250. DOI: 10.1002/14651858.CD012250.pub2

[22] Huo ZC, Liu G, Li XY, Liu F, Fan WJ, Guan RH, et al. Use of a disposable circumcision suture device versus conventional circumcision: A systematic review and meta-analysis. Asian Journal of Andrology. 2017;**19**(3):362-367. DOI: 10.4103/1008-682X.174855

[23] Weiss HA, Larke N, Halperin D, Schenker I. Complications of circumcision in male neonates, infants and children: A systematic review. BMC Urology. 2010;**10**:2. DOI: 10.1186/1471-2490-10-2

[24] Tucker SC, Cerqueiro J, Sterne GD, Bracka A. Circumcision: A refined technique and 5 year review. Annals of the Royal College of Surgeons of England. 2001;**83**(2):121-125

[25] Okeke LI, Asinobi AA, Ikuerowo OS. Epidemiology of complications of Abdulwahab-Ahmed and Mungadi: Techniques of male circumcision journal of surgical technique and case report|Jan-Jun 2013, 5, 1, 7 male circumcision in Ibadan, Nigeria. BMC Urology. 2006;**6**:21

[26] Gee WF, Ansell JS. Neonatal circumcision: A ten-year overview: With comparison of the Gomco clamp and the Plastibell device. Pediatrics. 1976;**58**(6):824-827

[27] Kaplan GW. Complications of circumcision. The Urologic Clinics of North America. 1983;**10**(3):543-549

[28] Sterenberg N, Golan J, Ben-Hur N. Necrosis of the glans penis following neonatal circumcision. Plastic and Reconstructive Surgery. 1981;**68**(2):237-239. DOI: 10.1097/00006534-198108000-00022

[29] Senel FM, Demirelli M, Misirlioglu F, Sezgin T. Adult male circumcision performed with plastic clamp technique in Turkey: Results and long-term effects on sexual function. Urology Journal. 2012;**9**(4):700-705

Chapter 4

Laser Circumcision: A New Technique

Rosario Leonardi and Giuseppe Saitta

Abstract

In this chapter, we would like to enlighten the importance of circumcision as a feasible and sometimes necessary surgical technique. In particular, laser circumcision seems to be more effective than other minimally invasive techniques in terms of safety, reproducibility of the technique, learning curve, and reduced execution times. Moreover, it is associated with low rates of all circumcision complications: no bleeding, no postoperative edema, and rapid functional recovery. The aesthetic results are very pleasing.

Keywords: laser circumcision, safe, quickly, aesthetic, cost-effectiveness, reproducible, no complications, fast recovery

1. Introduction

Male circumcision consists of the surgical removal of some or all of the foreskin (or prepuce) from the penis. It is one of the most common procedures in the world. Moreover, specific benefits from this procedure were identified for the prevention of urinary tract infections, acquisition of HIV, transmission of some sexually transmitted infections, and penile cancer [1].

Some trials in Africa have demonstrated that adult MC decreases human immunodeficiency virus (HIV) acquisition by 51–60% in men, and also increased protection as it affects time after surgery [2].

Other ones showed that MC reduces the risk of other heterosexually acquired sexually transmitted infections (STIs): the risk of acquiring genital herpes by 28–34%, risk of developing genital ulceration by 47%.

Moreover, MC reduces the risk of oncogenic high-risk human papillomavirus (HR-HPV) by 32–35% [3].

Neonatal MC provides other potential benefits during childhood, such as prevention of infant urinary tract infections, meatitis, balanitis, phimosis, and also protection from viral STIs [4].

It is associated also with a lower prevalence of human papillomavirus (HPV) infection and herpes simplex virus-type 2 (HSV-2) transmission, and decreased rates of bacterial vaginosis (BV) in female partners with good evidence [5–8].

A meta-analysis found 68% lower balanitis rates after MC [9].

A large Australian survey reported penile candidiasis in 7.7% of uncircumcised men versus 4.9% of circumcised men [10].

The prevalence of fungal infection was 44% in uncircumcised boys versus 18% in circumcised boys [11].

Uncircumcised men had a 22-fold higher risk of penile cancer, according to a Californian study [12].

Countries with high MC prevalence have lower prostate cancer-related mortality, corrected for potential confounding factors [13].

Arguments opposing MC are supported mostly by low-quality evidence and opinion, and are contradicted by strong scientific evidence [14].

MC did not affect sexual dysfunction: In the trial from Kenya, 99.5% of circumcised participants reported that they were "very satisfied" for increased penile sensitivity. The vast majority of female partners of male participants in this trial reported that they were very satisfied (92%) or somewhat satisfied (5%) with the outcome of circumcision [15].

Circumcision may result in early (intraoperative) or late (postoperative) complications. Early complications are often minor and treatable: Bleeding, pain, swelling, or inadequate skin removal. Major complications, such as amputation of the glans or of the penis, occur very rarely. Persistent pain, wound infection, edema, urinary retention, meatal ulcer, meatal stenosis, foreskin adhesions, fistulas, and loss of penile sensitivity could be considered as late complications.

The complications rates may appear consistently divergent between the considered studies for various surgical procedures and also by different data collection methods [16].

2. Different techniques of circumcision

The three most common operative methods of circumcision are: the Gomco clamp, the plastibell device, and the Mogen clamp (or some variations) [1].

2.1 Gomco clamp

The Gomco clamp was specifically developed for performing MC.

In this procedure, "the foreskin is cut lengthwise through the stretched tissue to allow space in order to insert the device. The bell of the Gomco clamp is placed over the glans, and the foreskin is pulled over the bell. The base of the Gomco clamp is placed over the bell, and the Gomco clamp's arm is fitted. When the surgeon is sure of the correct fitting and placement by the amount of foreskin to be excised, the nut on the Gomco clamp is tightened and left in place for some minutes to obtain hemostasis, so the foreskin is removed using a scalpel."

Therefore the Gomco's base and bell are removed [17].

Some studies showed evidence of lower complication rates in newborn circumcisions, using this technique: an overall complication rate of 1.9% in Saudi Arabia, bleeding in 0.6%, infection in 0.4%, and redundant prepuce in 0.3% of cases.

Another one from Houston, including 521 newborn MC, showed a 2.9% incidence of phimosis (trapped penis) [18].

2.2 Plastibell device

In this circumcision, a plastic ring is inserted under the foreskin, and support is placed over the ring allowing hemostasis. The ring is left up on the penis for some days until tissue necrosis and spontaneous fall off the ring.

Studies on this device reported an overall complications rate from 2.4 to 5%, urinary retention in 3.6%, infections in 2.1%, and bleeding in 0.8–3% of cases [19–24].

2.3 Mogen clamp

This device consists of two flat blades that have limited space between them and a mechanism that draws the blades together and locks them in place. The slit is limited to 3 mm to allow the foreskin ride, but not the glans to cross the opening by the clamp. The foreskin is taken down and the glans pushed downward, protected from the blades. The prepuce distal to the glans is drawn into the slit between the blades and these are locked together, in order to push the skin and permit hemostasis. So, the skin is excised from above the clamp and the device is removed. Complications are rare [23–29].

3. Newborn circumcision techniques

In the last years, many authors have considered the possibility to perform MC with other new devices or maybe other newborn techniques, to reduce or even remove the time for sutures and hemostasis.

A systematic review containing eight RCTs and including 3314 patients, compared the safety and efficacy of traditional versus device-assisted circumcision, showing lower complication rates in the device group compared with the conventional technique group (RR 0.54, 95% CI 0.39–0.74): this difference was due in particular by higher healing and lower bleeding rates [30].

Contraindications to newborn circumcision include significantly premature infants, blood dyscrasias, family history of bleeding disorders, and those who have congenital abnormalities, such as hypospadias, congenital chordee, or deficient shaft skin, such as penoscrotal fusion or congenital buried penis [31].

The true incidence of complications after newborn circumcision is unknown, due to different definitions of "complications" and for the undetermined time of the problem appearing (i.e., early or late).

Adding to the confusion is the comingling of "early" complications, such as bleeding or infection, with "late" complications, such as adhesions and meatal stenosis.

The risk of significant acute MC complications by two large US studies was shown between 0.19% and 0.22%: bleeding from 0.08% to 0.18%, infection (0.06%), and penile injury (0.04%) [32–34].

The most common surgical complication is excessive bleeding (e.g., bleeding that did not stop with local pressure, perhaps requiring a suture), reported in 0.6% of 1742 male infants [35].

Late complications of newborn circumcision include excessive residual skin (incomplete circumcision), excessive skin removal, adhesions (natural and vascularized skin bridges), meatal stenosis, phimosis, and epithelial inclusion cysts.

Hohlfield et al. did not find serious difference between circumcision devices and surgical techniques [36].

There are many newborn techniques, but the most common provide the use of glues and bipolar energy.

3.1 Glue

Sutureless circumcision with tissue glue (iso amyl 2-cyanoacrylate) was cosmetically superior and timeless in comparison to traditional technique in Tiwari's Indian experience [37].

The glue was comparatively safe, efficient, and had a better functional outcome and good cosmesis in the comparative study by Raut [38].

Histoacryl glue saved operative time and was associated with less postoperative pain (severity and duration) [39].

3.2 Bipolar

The bipolar scissors circumcision approach was an effective and safe procedure alternative to the standard scalpel technique in pediatric circumcision with no significant morbidity [40].

This technique was safe and achieved good cosmetic results [41].

The use of bipolar diathermy was shown to be simple, safe, and acceptable [42, 43].

4. Laser circumcision

The carbon dioxide laser for circumcision was introduced in 1989 by the Department of Pediatric Surgery, KK Women's & Children's Hospital in Singapore [44].

In 2004 Vaos compared the clinical effects of the Nd:YAG laser contact technique with those of a conventional technique on the grounds of certain perioperative parameters, including operative time, length of hospital stay, postoperative complications, and morbidity. Thinking that the tissue effects of the Nd:YAG laser contact technique theoretically may attenuate some of the causes of postoperative complications, he demonstrated an effective laser-assisted procedure as a valid alternative to the conventional technique in circumcision with no significant postoperative morbidity [45].

In 2020 an Italian study wished to evaluate the benefits of the use of carbon dioxide (CO_2) laser versus the conventional procedure for circumcision in adults, in terms of duration of surgery, surgical techniques, complications, pain, and cosmetic appearance. So, they showed that the use of a CO_2 laser was associated with a shorter operative time, less wound irritation, and better cosmetic appearance compared with standard surgical techniques for circumcision [46].

We performed 22 laser circumcisions (10/15 W, 1470 nm, 600 μ) with good results [*].

Table 1 resumes the results shown by some authors in terms of functional outcomes (pain, bleeding, edema, and fast recovery), operation time, and good cosmesis between different circumcision techniques: traditional surgery, glue, bipolar, and lasers.

4.1 Safety

Laser circumcision (LC) appears as a safe and reproducible procedure with few complications, almost no bleeding, and no postoperative edema and inflammation.

Circumcision studies	Functional outcomes (in terms of pain, bleeding, edema, fast recovery)	Operation time (min)	Good cosmesis
Traditional			
[36]	more pain at 24 hours, no difference at 7 days	24	—
[37]	no significative difference	24.4 ± 5.06	—
[38]	—	—	excessive swelling
[39]	more postoperative pain	—	—
[40]	blood loss 2.1 ml (range, 0.9–4.2 mL)	19.1 ± 2.6	—
	22 patients with postoperative edema		
[45]	length of hospital stay 11.8 ± 5.1 h	19.8 ± 1.9	—
	early postoperative morbidity 9%		
	late postoperative morbidity 7.2%		
[46]	47 patients (27.9%) with pronounced edema	23.1 ± 2.8	103 patients (61.3%)
[47]	mean blood loss 7.2 + − 1.5 g, more pain at 1 and 7 days	21.1 ± 2.7	—
[48]	—	22 (20–26)	—
[49]	higher rate of local irritation	50.4	poor appearance
Glue			
[36]	lower pain at 24 hours, no difference at 7 days	17	—
[37]	no significative difference	—	—
[38]	—	14.2 ± 2.42	cosmetically superior
[39]	less postoperative pain	—	no swelling
[48]	—	7 (6–9)	—
[49]	lower rate of local irritation	30.8	all patients satisfied
Bipolar			
[40]	blood loss 0.2 ml (range, 0–0.8 mL)	10.8 ± 1.2	—
	10 patients with postoperative edema		
[41]	—	—	satisfactory quantified
[42]	1/30 patients	—	all patients satisfied
Laser			
[45] Nd:YAG	length of hospital stay 9.71 ± 4.5 h	31.6 ± 3.6	—
	early postoperative morbidity 2%		
	late postoperative morbidity 0%		
[46] CO2	62 (19.7%) with pronounced edema	12.8 ± 0.9	298 patients (94.9%)
[*]	no early postoperative morbidity	15.6 ± 5.2	all patients satisfied
[47] CO2	no blood loss, less pain at 1 and 7 days	10.5 ± 0.9	—
[48] CO2	—	7 (6–9)	—
[49] CO2	lower rate of local irritation	30.8	all patients satisfied

no significative difference: p value >0.05.
—: no information about.

Table 1.
Comparative data between different circumcision techniques.

The purpose of the study conducted by Xu et al. was to investigate the safety and efficacy of a modified CO_2 laser technique for circumcision in adult males as compared with the conventional dorsal-slit method. A total of 300 patients >18 years of age were recruited for this study. Several perioperative data, including age, indications, operation time, intraoperative blood loss, complications, and postoperative pain, were analyzed. With respect to blood loss, there was almost no blood loss during the operation using the CO_2 laser, whereas the mean blood loss was 7.2 + − 1.5 g in the conventional group ($p < 0.05$). The CO_2 laser technique was associated with less pain at 1 day (2.9 + − 1.9 vs. 4.9 + − 2.5, $p < 0.05$) and 7 days postoperatively (1.2 + − 0.5 vs. 1.9 + − 1.3, $p < 0.05$) [47].

Huang et al. found the use of Holmium YAG laser in circumcision as a novel, less complicated, easy, and less painful alternative procedure for circumcision in young males [50].

Patients have a risk of complications, such as local edema and tenderness, scarring, wound dehiscence, hematoma, and infections, despite the fact that MC is largely considered a minor surgical procedure [51–53].

It was demonstrated that the Holmium:YAG is effective for the treatment of soft tissue pathologies, for example, BPE/BPO, upper tract urothelial carcinomas (UTUC), and urinary strictures. The Holmium:YAG laser has strong absorption of water molecules around 2140 nm, which implies a short destruction length in the tissue [50].

Carbon oxide lasers are currently widely used to perform MC, for the following positive features: CO_2 laser procures good incision and hemostasis because a high-power setting can cauterize small vessels; the incision is more effective with a CO_2 laser compared to the traditional scalpel method; patients feel less postoperative pain and declare more comfort.

These facts are corroborated by several studies. The lower postoperative complication rate in the laser group compared to the conventional group was showed by Xu et al.: less bleeding and shorter operative times [47].

Another important question discussed is the potential sub-clinical injury by electrosurgery on the penile tissue. Conventional monopolar electrocoagulation may cause electrical burns, necrosis, and penile damage [54–58].

An experiment by Tsai et al. demonstrated that the electrical field strength of the whole penis shaft was 9.03 V/cm, so it was found heat generated from the penis is four times that of other body parts, which may contribute to erectile tissue damage. Therefore, new laser technologies, including CO_2, Nd-YAG, or Holmium:YAG laser, are considered superior methods after the conduction of this study [59].

4.2 Fast surgery

LC needs not too much experience to have good results (we could talk about "learning curve", although there are no major studies on this in the literature).

It is associated with reduced operative times, fast recovery, and quick return to normal life.

A comparison of the patients in the two groups of the Chinese study demonstrated a 10 minutes decrease in the operative time in the laser-treated group (10.5 + −0.9 vs. 21.1 + −2.7 min, $p < 0.05$) [47].

There was a significant decrease of 5 minutes in operating time for the group of patients who underwent laser circumcision in the retrospective review by the Singapore group of pediatric surgery [44].

Vaos highlighted increased operative time in the Nd:YAG laser group compared with the group of patients treated by conventional technique (31.6 ± 3.6 min vs. 19.8 ± 1.9 min, $p < 0.001$), reduced rates of early and late postoperative complications (2% vs. 9%, $p < 0.05$ and 0% vs. 7.2%, $p < 0.05$, respectively) and also reduced length of hospital stay in comparison with the traditional technique (9.71 ± 4.5 h vs. 11.8 ± 5.1 h, $p < 0.05$) [45].

Gorgulu et al. developed a combined technique with CO2 laser and cyanoacrylate in order to prevent hematoma and hemorrhage, so in their results, they had a short operation median time (7 minutes vs. 22 minutes of the conventional guillotine group) [48].

4.3 Aesthetic results

LC represents an aesthetically satisfying technique, maybe better of the traditional one.

Thirty boys were divided into two groups in the study by Mungnirandr et al.: Group 1 (n = 17) underwent MC by scalpel and approximation of the wound edges by sutures. Group 2 (n = 13) underwent circumcision with CO2 laser and approximation of the wound edges using tissue glue.

The following parameters were recorded: patient age, indications for surgery, operation time, wound bleeding, swelling or infection, pain, local irritation, and cosmetic result.

Only one case of bleeding was reported in Group 1.

Group 2 showed a shorter operative time ($p = 0.011$), lower rate of local irritation ($p = 0.016$), and better aesthetic picture ($p < 0.001$) than Group 1.

CO2 laser and tissue glue have advantages over standard surgical techniques in circumcision, with a significantly shorter operative time, lower rate of local irritation, and better cosmetic appearance. There were no significant differences in pain score, wound infection rate, or cost of surgery between the two groups [49].

Lichen sclerosus (LS) is a chronic inflammatory skin disease that primarily affects the anogenital region. The disease can affect patients of all ages, in particular in the fifth or sixth decade, but it is rare in children. Etiology is unknown, maybe in genetically predisposed patients, an important pathogenetic role could be represented by the immune system. LS often plays with a relapsing trend that can lead to scars, cutaneous atrophy, and functional impairment [60].

LS is associated with an increased risk of developing spinous cell carcinoma in the affected genital area. Chronic irritation, trauma, and occlusion under the prepuce represent precipitating factors [61].

Some researchers carried out treatments using a fractional micro-ablative CO2 laser (SmartXide2, DEKA, M.E.L.A, Florence, Italy), with these parameters: emission mode, high pulse (HP); power, 10–13 W; spacing between dots, 500 and 600 μm; the number of pulses on the same spot, 1–2. They repeated the treatment at a monthly interval till achieving good clinical and aesthetic results, so five sessions were necessary to obtain an excellent outcome [60].

The figures below show some cosmetic results obtained with our laser technique.

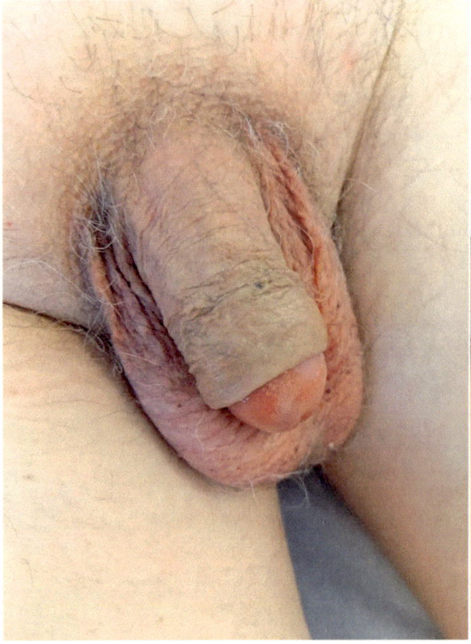

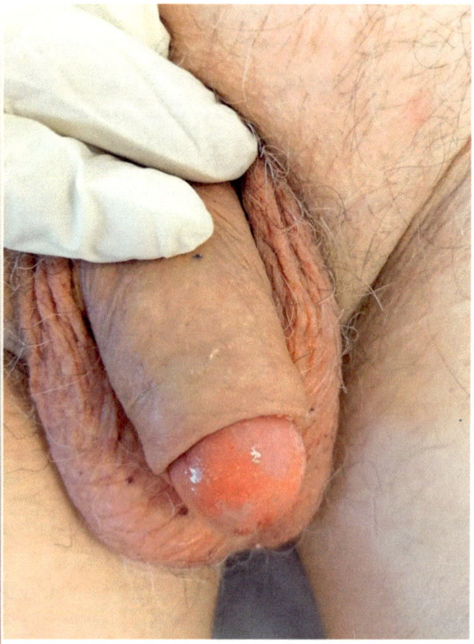

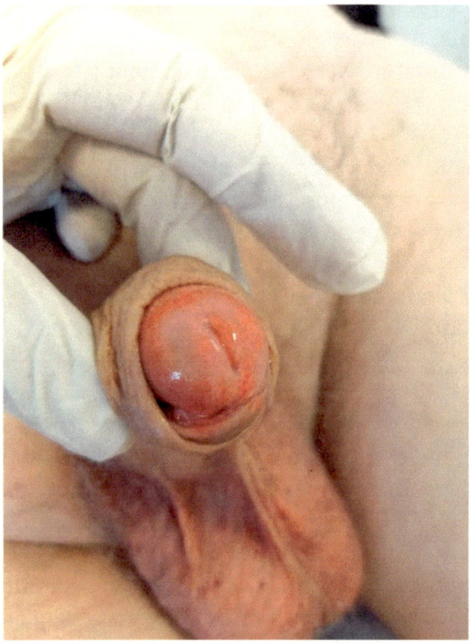

4.4 Costs

LC deserves low costs, especially when compared to other techniques (traditional and non-traditional).

In 2001 How et al. carried out a retrospective study comparing the operative times of two groups of 30 patients both: the first ones underwent conventional circumcision in 1985 and the other ones were treated in 1995 by LC.

The total cost of use of the laser machine was calculated, considering maintenance costs, estimated life span of the machines (10 years), and disposables used during each procedure. This was counted against the cost savings from shorter operating times and operating room facilities. Furthermore, morbidity data from 2781 LC performed between May 1997 and April 2000 were collected.

Calculated cost savings per laser circumcision from the reduced operating theater time was S$31/–.

There was an overall complication rate of 1.15%, related to the 2781 LC. Bleeding occurred in 29 patients (1.04%), of which 10 cases (0.36%) required to return to the operating theater for hemostasis. Wound infection requiring readmission to the hospital was described in three cases (0.11% of cases).

LC represents a simple technique with reduced operative time and consequently cost-effectiveness. Complication rates of laser circumcision compared to those of conventional circumcision appear favorable [44].

There are also some studies considering the savings attributed to the reduction of HIV infection by circumcision procedures. Kacker et al. assessed that continued decreases in MC rates are associated with increased infection prevalence [62].

5. Circumcision and COVID-19

Since the COVID-19 pandemic has widespread around the world, we should also consider all the medical, legal, and economic aspects related to the new situation.

Healthcare lockdown involving the cancelation or postponement of nonurgent examinations and treatments during the pandemic has reduced the number of emergency department visits by urological patients. Of the most common urological procedure types, the lockdown had a clear negative effect on the incidence of BPO, as well as foreskin excision procedure [63, 64].

The laser technique does not require any anesthesia or only a local one, so the patient can keep well the mask during the procedure, reducing the risk of infecting and being infected, especially in cases where a PCR-test is not performed before the circumcision procedure. (e.g., outpatient procedure).

Rivera-Calonje et al. reported a case of COVID-19 positive 12 years old patient who presented for urgent wound incision and drainage at the circumcision site. He was transported from the COVID-19 isolation floor to the negative pressure operating room. He was placed in a lateral decubitus position and oxygen was delivered through a facemask. Under sedation, spinal anesthesia was achieved at the first attempt as a safe alternative to general endotracheal anesthesia [65].

6. Conclusions

For all the reasons explained we believe that laser use may become the gold standard of circumcision in the next future or in any case be more considered than traditional surgery and maybe also than newborn techniques.

Conflict of interest

"The authors declare no conflict of interest."

Abbreviations

AAP:	American Academy of Pediatrics
BPE:	Benign Prostatic Enlargement
BPO:	Benign Prostatic Obstruction
BV:	Bacterial Vaginosis
CDC:	Centers for Disease Control and Prevention
CI:	Confidence Interval
CO2:	Carbon Dioxide
COVID:	Corona Virus Disease
HIV:	Human Immunodeficiency Virus
HoLEP:	Holmium Laser Enucleation Prostate
HP:	High Pulse
HPV:	Human Papillomavirus
HR:	High-Risk
HSV:	Herpes Simplex Virus
IELT:	Intravaginal Ejaculatory Latency Times
LC:	Laser Circumcision
LS:	Lichen Sclerosus
MC:	Male Circumcision
Nd:YAG:	Neodymium-Doped Yttrium Aluminum Garnet
PCR:	Polymerase Chain Reaction
OR:	Odds Ratio
RCT:	Randomized Controlled Trial
STI:	Sexually Transmitted Infection
US:	United States
UTI:	Urinary Tract Infection
UTUC:	Upper Tract Urothelial Carcinoma
V:	Volume
W:	Watt

Author details

Rosario Leonardi[1] and Giuseppe Saitta[2*]

1 Musumeci GECAS Clinic, Gravina di Catania, Italy

2 IRCCS Istituto Auxologico Italiano, Milano, Italy

*Address all correspondence to: gsaitta@hotmail.it

References

[1] Male Circumcision. Technical Report of American Academy of Pediatrics www.pediatrics.org/cgi/doi/10.1542/peds.2012-1990

[2] Tobian AAR, Gray RH. The medical benefits of male circumcision. Journal of the American Medical Association. 2011;**306**(13):1479-1480. DOI: 10.1001/jama.2011.1431

[3] Tobian AA, Gray RH, Quinn TC. Male circumcision for the prevention of acquisition and transmission of sexually transmitted infections: The case for neonatal circumcision. Archives of Pediatrics & Adolescent Medicine. 2010;**164**(1):78-84 [PubMed: 20048246]

[4] American Academy of Pediatrics Task Force on Circumcision. Circumcision policy statement. Pediatrics. 1999;**103**(3):686-693 [PubMed: 10049981]

[5] Sexually transmitted diseases (STDs): genital herpes. CDC Fact Sheet. Atlanta, GA: Centers for Disease Control and Prevention; 2012. Available at: www.cdc.gov/std/herpes/stdfact-herpes.htm

[6] Wawer MJ, Tobian AA, Kigozi G, et al. Effect of circumcision of HIV-negative men on transmission of human papillomavirus to HIV-negative women: A randomised trial in Rakai, Uganda. Lancet. 2011;**377**(9761):209-218

[7] Cherpes TL, Meyn LA, Krohn MA, Hillier SL. Risk factors for infection with herpes simplex virus type 2: Role of smoking, douching, uncircumcised males, and vaginal flora. Sexually Transmitted Diseases. 2003;**30**(5):405-410

[8] Sexually transmitted diseases: bacterial vaginosis. CDC Fact Sheet. Atlanta, GA: Centers for Disease Control and Prevention; 2010 Available at: www.cdc.gov/std/bv/STDFact-Bacterial-Vaginosis.htm

[9] Morris BJ, Gray RH, Castellsague X, et al. The strong protective effect of circumcision against cancer of the penis. Advances Urology. 2011;**2011**:812368

[10] Ferris JA, Richters J, Pitts MK, et al. Circumcision in Australia: Further evidence on its effects on sexual health and wellbeing. Australian and New Zealand Journal of Public Health. 2010;**34**:160-164

[11] Iskit S, Ilkit M, Turc-Bicer A, Demirhindi H, Turker M. Effect of circumcision on genital colonization of Malassezia spp. in a pediatric population. Medical Mycology. 2006;**44**:113-117

[12] Schoen EJ, Oehrli M, Colby C, Machin G. The highly protective effect of newborn circumcision against invasive penile cancer. Pediatrics. 2000;**105**:E36

[13] Wachtel MS, Yang S, Morris BJ. Countries with high circumcision prevalence have lower prostate cancer mortality. Asian Journal of Andrology. 2016;**18**:39-42

[14] Morris BJ, Moreton S, Krieger JN. Critical evaluation of arguments opposing male circumcision: A systematic review. Journal of Evidence-Based Medicine. 2019;**12**:263-290. DOI: 10.1111/jebm.12361

[15] Krieger JN, Bailey RC, Opeya JC, Ayieko BO, Opiyo FA, Omondi D, et al. Adult male circumcision outcomes: Experience in a developing country setting. Urologia Internationalis. 2007;**78**:235-240

[16] Friedman B, Khoury J, Petersiel N, Yahalomi T, Paul M, Neuberger A. Pros and cons of circumcision: An evidence-based overview. Clinical Microbiology and Infection. 2016;**22**:768-774

[17] Wikipedia. Gomco Clamp. Available at: http://en.wikipedia.org/wiki/Gomco_clamp#cite_note-8

[18] Blalock HJ, Vemulakonda V, Ritchey ML, Ribbeck M. Outpatient management of phimosis following newborn circumcision. The Journal of Urology. 2003;**169**(6):2332-2334

[19] Manji KP. Circumcision of the young infant in a developing country using the Plastibell. Annals of Tropical Paediatrics. 2000;**20**(2):101-104

[20] Mihssin N, Moorthy K, Houghton PW. Retention of urine: An unusual complication of the Plastibell device. BJU International. 1999;**84**(6):745

[21] Bliss DP, Healey PJ, Waldhausen JH. Necrotizing fasciitis after Plastibell circumcision. The Journal of Pediatrics. 1997;**131**(3):459-462

[22] Palit V, Menebhi DK, Taylor I, Young M, Elmasry Y, Shah T. A unique service in UK delivering Plastibell circumcision: Review of 9-year results. Pediatric Surgery International. 2007;**23**(1):45-48

[23] Duncan ND, Dundas SE, Brown B, Pinnock Ramsaran C, Badal G. Newborn circumcision using the Plastibell device: An audit of practice. The West Indian Medical Journal. 2004;**53**(1):23-26

[24] Lazarus J, Alexander A, Rode H. Circumcision complications associated with the Plastibell device. South African Medical Journal. 2007;**97**(3):192-193

[25] Beniamin F, Castagnetti M, Rigamonti W. Surgical management of penile amputation in children. Journal of Pediatric Surgery. 2008;**43**:1939-1943

[26] de Lagausie P, Jehanno P. Six years followup of a penis replantation in a child. Journal of Pediatric Surgery. 2008;**43**:E11-E12

[27] Perovic SV, Djinovic RP, Bumbasirevic MZ, Santucci RA, Djordjevic ML, Kourbatov D. Severe penile injuries: A problem of severity and reconstruction. BJU International. 2009;**104**:676-687

[28] Shaeer O. Restoration of the penis following amputation at circumcision: Shaeer's AY plasty. The Journal of Sexual Medicine. 2008;**5**:1013-1021

[29] Binous MY, Haddad B, Fekih W, Boudokhane M, Hellali K, Fodha M. Amputation of a penile glans distal third and successful reattachment. La Tunisie Médicale. 2008;**86**:608-609

[30] Cao D, Liu L, Hu Y, Wang J, Yuan J, Dong Q, et al. A systematic review and meta-analysis of circumcision with Shang ring vs conventional circumcision. Urology. 2015;**85**:799-804

[31] American Academy of Pediatrics Committee on Fetus and Newborn. Controversies concerning vitamin K and the newborn. Pediatrics. 2003;**112** (1 pt 1):191-192

[32] Christakis DA, Harvey E, Zerr DM, Feudtner C, Wright JA, Connell FA. A trade-off analysis of routine newborn circumcision. Pediatrics. 2000;**105** (1 pt 3):246-249

[33] Learman LA. Neonatal circumcision: a dispassionate analysis. Clinical Obstetrics and Gynecology. 1999;**42**(4):849-859

[34] Wiswell TE, Geschke DW. Risks from circumcision during the first

month of life compared with those for uncircumcised boys. Pediatrics. 1989;**83**(6):1011-1015

[35] O'Brien TR, Calle EE, Poole WK. Incidence of neonatal circumcision in Atlanta, 1985- 1986. Southern Medical Journal. 1995;**88**(4):411-415

[36] Hohlfiel ASJ, Ebrahim S, Shaik MZ, Kredo T. Circumcision devices versus standard surgical techniques in adolescent and adult male circumcisions: A Cochrane review. BJU International. 2021:4-5. DOI: 10.1111/bju.15604

[37] Tiwari P, Tiwari A, Kumar S, Rajkumar Patil2, Amit Goel, Pramod Sharma, Anup K. Kundu. Sutureless circumcision - an Indian experience. Indian. The Journal of Urology. 2011;**27**(4):475-478. DOI: 10.4103/0970-1591.91435

[38] Raut A. Sutureless versus sutured circumcision: A comparative study. Urology Annals. 2019;**11**(1):87-90. DOI: 10.4103/UA.UA_12_18

[39] Subramaniam R, Jacobsen AS. Sutureless circumcision: A prospective randomised controlled study. Pediatric Surgery International. 2004;**20**(10):783-785. DOI: 10.1007/s00383-004-1149-z

[40] Méndez-Gallart R, Estévez E, Bautista A, Rodríguez P, Taboada P, Armas AL, et al. Bipolar scissors circumcision is a safe, fast, and bloodless procedure in children. Journal of Pediatric Surgery. OPERATIVE TECHNIQUE. 2009;**44**(10):2048-2053. DOI: 10.1016/j.jpedsurg.2009.06.008

[41] El-Mefleh N, Kaddah M, Ba'Ath ME. Bipolar circumcision: A new technique for an old procedure with quantified cosmetic outcome. African Journal of Paediatric Surgery. 2021;**18**(4):187-189. DOI: 10.4103/ajps.AJPS_108_20

[42] Fraser I, Tjoe J. Circumcision using bipolar diathermy scissors. A simple, safe and acceptable technique. Annals of the Royal College of Surgeons of England. 2000;**82**:190-191

[43] Fraser ID, Goede AC. Sutureless circumcision. POINT OF TECHNIQUE. BJU International. 2002;**90**:467-468

[44] How ACSW, Ong CCP, Jacobsen A, Joseph VT. Carbon dioxide laser circumcisions for children. Pediatric Surgery International. 2003;**19**(1-2):11-13. DOI: 10.1007/s00383-002-0894-0 Epub 2003 Jan 9

[45] Vaos G. Circumcision with the Nd:YAG laser contact technique compared with conventional surgery. Photomedicine and Laser Surgery. 2004;**22**(4):318-322. DOI: 10.1089/pho.2004.22.318

[46] Ronchi P, Manno S, Lucio D'A. Technology meets tradition: CO2 laser circumcision versus conventional surgical technique. Research and Reports in Urology. 2020;**12**:255-260

[47] Yansheng X, Li F, Li Z, Guan W, Yiguang W, Ouyang Y, et al. A prospective, randomized controlled trial of circumcision in adult males using the CO2 laser: Modified technique compared with the conventional dorsal-slit technique. Photomedicine and Laser Surgery. 2013;**31**(9):422-427. DOI: 10.1089/pho.2013.3550 Epub 2013 Jul 20

[48] Gorgulu T, Olgun A, Torun M, Kargi E. A fast, easy circumcision procedure combining a CO2 laser and cyanoacrylate adhesive: A non-randomized comparative trial. International Braz J Urol. 2016;**42**(1):113-117. DOI: 10.1590/S1677-5538.IBJU.2015.0284

[49] Mungnirandr A, Wiriyakamolphan S, Ruangtrakool R, Ngerncham M,

Tumrongsombutsakul S, Leumcharoen B. Comparison of a CO2 (carbon dioxide) laser and tissue glue with conventional surgical techniques in circumcision. Journal of lasers in medical sciences Winter. 2015;**6**(1):28-37

[50] Huang P-L, Lee I-C, Tsai D-C, Tsai J-H, Tsai VFS, Pong Y-H. Use of holmium YAG laser in circumcision: A novel, less complicated and alternative procedure for adolescent. Huang et al. The African Journal of Urology. 2020;**26**:64. DOI: 10.1186/s12301-020-00077-y

[51] Krill AJ, Palmer LS, Palmer JS. Complications of circumcision. Scientific World Journal. 2011;**11**:2458-2468

[52] Weiss HA, Larke N, Halperin D, et al. Complications of circumcision in male neonates, infants and children: A systematic review. BMC Urology. 2010;**10**:2

[53] Barrier G, Attia J, Mayer MN, et al. Measurement of post-operative pain and narcotic administration in infants using a new clinical scoring system. Intensive Care Medicine. 1989;**15**(Suppl. 1):S37-S39

[54] Gearhart JP, Rock JA. Total ablation of the penis after circumcision with electrocautery: A method of management and long-term followup. The Journal of Urology. 1989;**142**:799-801

[55] Hsu GL, Hsieh CH, Wen HS, et al. The efect of electrocoagulation on the sinusoids in the human penis. Journal of Andrology. 2004;**25**:954-959

[56] Seleim HM, Elbarbary MM. Major penile injuries as a result of cautery during newborn circumcision. Journal of Pediatric Surgery. 2016;**51**:1532-1537

[57] Uzun G, Ozdemir Y, Eroglu M, et al. Electrocautery-induced Gan- grene of the glans penis in a child following circumcision. BML Case Reports. 2012;**2012**:1

[58] Song LJ, Zhu JQ, Xie MK, et al. Electrocautery-induced cavernous nerve injury in rats that mimics radical prostatectomy in humans. BJU International. 2014;**114**:133-139

[59] Tsai VF, Chang HC, Liu SP, et al. Determination of human penile electrical resistance and implication on safety for electrosurgery of penis. The Journal of Sexual Medicine. 2010;**7**:2891-2898

[60] Campolmi P, Cannarozzo G, Bennardo L, Clementi A, Sannino M, Nisticò SP. Fractional micro-ablative CO2 laser as therapy in penile lichen Sclerosus. Journal of Lasers in Medical Sciences. 2021;**12**:e61, 2021. DOI: 10.34172/jlms.2021.61. eCollection

[61] Fistarol SK, Itin PH. Diagnosis and treatment of lichen sclerosus: An update. American Journal of Clinical Dermatology. 2013;**14**(1):27-47. DOI: 10.1007/s40257-012-0006-4

[62] Kacker S, Frick KD, Gaydos CA, Tobian AAR. Costs and effectiveness of neonatal male circumcision. Archives of Pediatrics & Adolescent Medicine. 2012;**166**(10):910-918. DOI: 10.1001/archpediatrics.2012.1440

[63] Gallioli A, Albo G, Lievore E, et al. How the COVID-19 wave changed emergency urology: Results from an academic tertiary referral hospital in the epicentre of the Italian red zone. Urology. 2021;**147**:43-49

[64] Grasso AA, Massa G, Castelnuovo M. The impact of COVID-19 pandemic on urological emergencies: A multicenter experience on over 3,000 patients. Urologia Internationalis. 2021;**105**:17-20

[65] Rivera-Calonje F, Chen SE, Lo C, Le S, Nagoshi M. Urgent surgery for COVID-19-positive pediatric patient. JA Clinical Reports. 2021;**7**(1):57. DOI: 10.1186/s40981-021-00461-9

Section 3

Periprocedural Analgesia

Chapter 5

Circumcision with Thermocautery after Local Anesthesia in Children: A Retrospective Single-Center Experience

Mehmet Uysal

Abstract

This study aimed to examine the short- and long-term complications of thermocautery-assisted circumcisions with local anesthesia done in a sterile environment in operating room conditions, accompanied by literature. The participants who consecutively underwent thermocautery-assisted circumcision with local anesthesia from June 2018 to May 2019 were included in the study. As a local anesthetic, 40-mg lidocaine HCl, 0.025-mg adrenaline, and bupivacaine 5 mg/ml were used together. They were 1 month to 17 years old, had same ethnic origin, and were in the same location. The age groups were compared in terms of complications. The participant age and surgical duration means were 4.89 ± 2.08 (30 days to 17 years) years old and 7.484 ± 1.524 (5–20 min) min, respectively. Complications were observed in 53 participants or 2.9% of the whole observation set. The participants under intervals of 1–6 months and over 6 years of age had significantly lower complication rates when compared to the other participants, and this comparison was statistically significant ($P = 0.001$). The study results demonstrated that circumcision with thermocautery after local anesthesia is a viable, reliable, and effective method. It can be assumed that circumcisions in males especially may be effective in 1–6 months and over 6 years of age. Parents choose this method because it is more appropriate and eliminates the risk of general anesthesia.

Keywords: bupivacaine, lidocaine, circumcision with local anesthesia

1. Introduction

Circumcision is a surgical procedure that means the removal of the foreskin from the male penis [1]. It is mostly performed for religious reasons in Turkey. In the Western Society, since the nineteenth century, circumcision began to be performed for medical reasons, and routine circumcision practice was abandoned in 1949 with the question of the medical benefits of circumcision [2, 3]. Regardless of the reason, one out of every six men in the world is circumcised [4, 5]. Apart from medical reasons, circumcision is performed to protect against sexually transmitted diseases

(STDs), as well as mostly for traditional and religious reasons [6, 7]. This surgical procedure is applied in almost every region of the world, although its frequency varies by region [8, 9]. Complications related to factors such as anatomical anomalies, clinical comorbidities, surgical methods used, and age of patients are seen in 1–4% of all the circumcision procedures. When circumcision is performed without sufficient experience and in inappropriate conditions, the risk of complications increases even more [7, 8]. Circumcision complications are categorized as early and late complications. Mild complications, such as pain, bleeding, edema, and inadequate skin excision, may occur in the early period, while infection, the formation of skin bridges, urinary retention, meatal stenosis, meatal ulcer, and fistulas can be examined in the late period [7, 10]. Indispensible challenges, such as death and glans amputation, may also appear, but rarely [11]. The medical basis of circumcision, when, where, and by whom, is not a complete opinion in the world, especially in Turkey.

2. Patients and methods

This research was performed in accordance with the Helsinki Declaration and with the approval of the local ethics committee (Clinical Ethics Committee of Karamanoğlu Mehmet Bey University Medical School, date 27.01.2021, issue 01.2021/01). This study was started with 2245 patients who were registered for

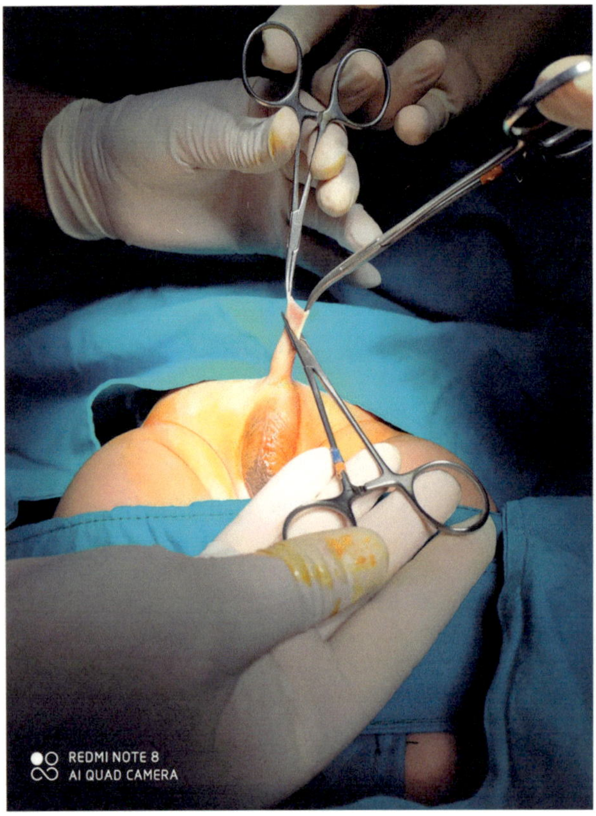

Figure 1.
Surgical step of thermocautery circumcision.

circumcision in our hospital's database, but 1821 patients who came for control on the 10th day, 1st month, and 1st year after circumcision were included.

The data of patients circumcised by pediatric surgery specialists between June 2018 and May 2019 were retrospectively restored and included in the study at the Karaman Training and Educational Hospital Pediatric Surgery Clinic in Turkey. Clinicians aged 1 month to 17 years who underwent circumcision with local anesthesia were included in this sampling retrospective study. The number of patients included in the study according to age groups was as follows: 30 days to 6 months: 630 (34.6%), 6–12 months: 358 (19.7%), 1–3 years: 152 (8.3%), 3–6 years: 54 (3%), and 6–17 years: 627 (34.4%). Patients who had existed simultaneously with diseases were excluded. In addition, consent forms were obtained from the legal representatives of the patients for the use of the medical images. The patients were recorded by local voluntary agencies before the date of circumcision. The labels consisted of the following sections: name, surname, birth date, birthplace, and previous disease. All the patients were examined prior to circumcision.

All the patients were carried out by one pediatric surgery specialist. As a local anesthetic, 40-mg lidocaine HCl, 0.025-mg adrenaline, and bupivacaine 5 mg/ml were used together. A penile block was imposed on the radix and circumference of the penis; 3–5 ml of local anesthetic was conducted according to the patients' age and weight. Regularly, the penis was cleaned with batticon and covered with a sterile surgical cover. Approximately 10 min after the injection of local anesthesia, the

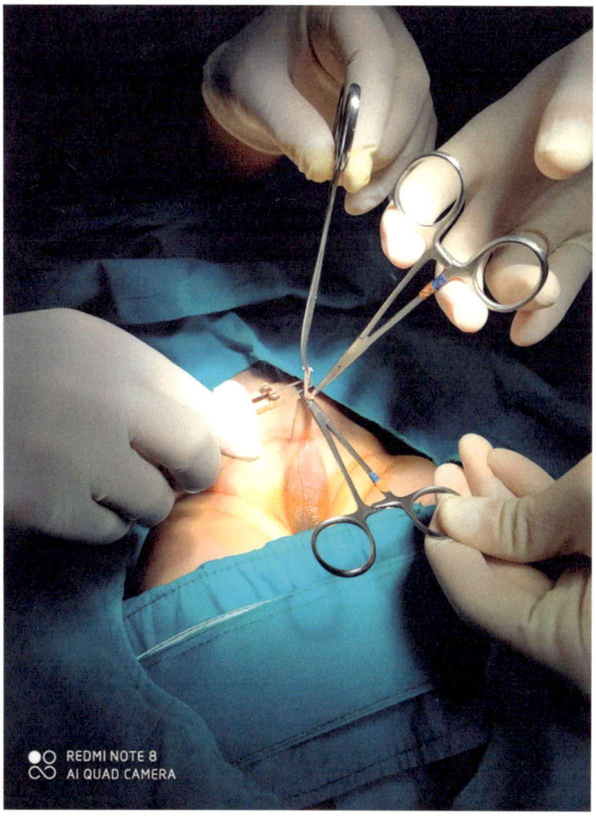

Figure 2.
Surgical step of thermocautery circumcision.

prepuce was pulled back to interfere with glans injury and the process was started, after observing and cleaning the external meatus and glans. The prepuce was covered using two clamps at positions 6 and 12 o'clock to design a slight strain and prepared the length of mucosa circumcised skin. It was established obliquely at an angle close to 15–20°, with its ventral part facing above. Thus, the meatus and frenulum were saved from injury. The guillotine technique was used in all the circumcisions performed with thermocautery included in our study. It is not recommended because it may cause glans incisions, but it is a method applied in current practice. In this method, after the prepuce is suspended with clamps, the surgeon pulls the glans down with the thumb and index finger of one hand and places the flat clamp on the prepuce in the other hand so that it is above the glans. The prepuce is cut with a scalpel over the clamp (**Figure 1**) Then, the mucosa is covered with clamps and the excess is excised (**Figure 2**). The skin and mucous membranes are sutured all around with separate sutures (**Figure 3**). In this method, it should be ensured that the glans remain under the clamp. Otherwise, there may be serious glans injuries [1]. The skin was covered and firmed on two sides by the clamp and foreskin tissue was cut just above the clamp (**Figure 2**) using a thermocautery device (Thermo-Med QX 2100; Thermo Medical, Adana, Turkey (**Figure 4**). The settings of the thermocautery device were set up according to the patient's age: 500°C was used for patients under 2 years of age; 550–650°C was used for patients of 2–10 years of age, and 700–750°C was used for patients older than 10 years of age. After bleeding was restrained, mucosal proportion

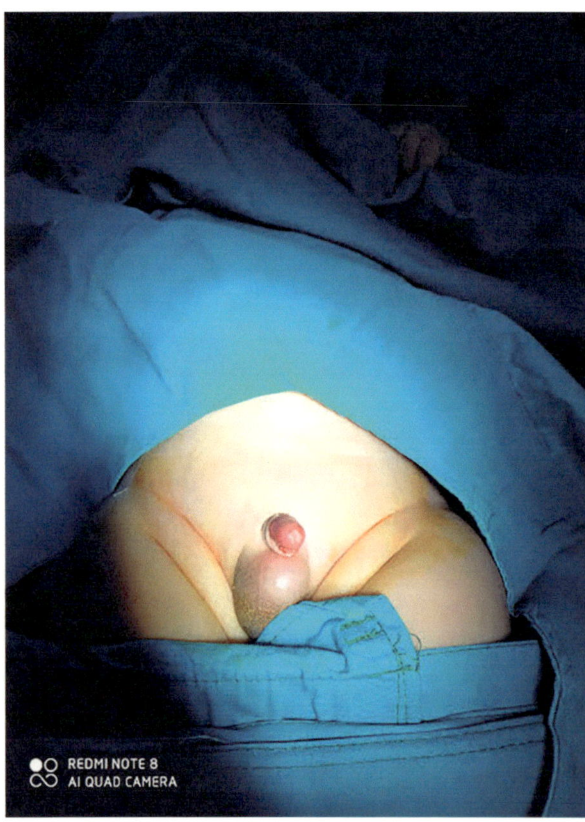

Figure 3.
Surgical step of thermocautery circumcision.

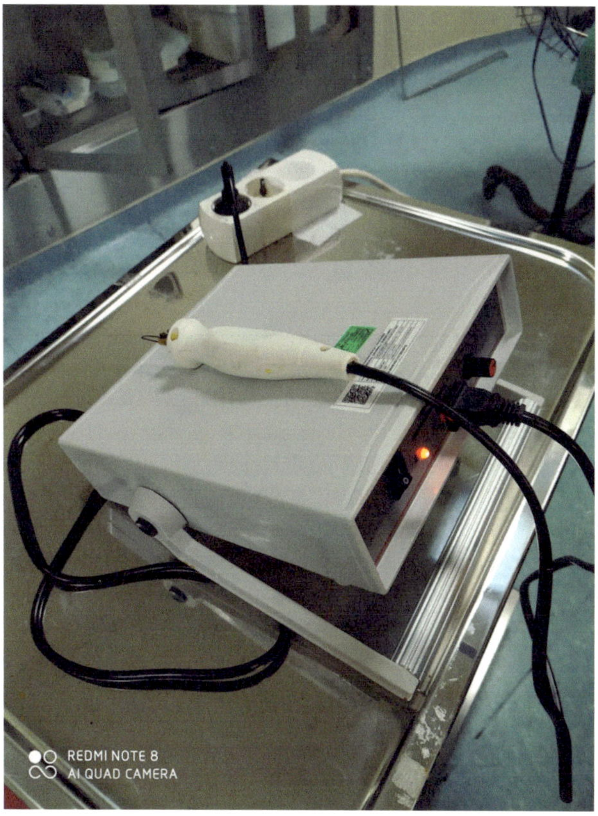

Figure 4.
Thermocautery device.

in patients under 2 years of age was supplied with two 5/0 absorbable sutures at 3, 6, 9, and 12 o'clock positions. A 4/0 absorbable suture was used in patients aged 2–10 years, with four sutures at 3, 5, 6, 7, 9, and 12 o'clock positions.

Finally, in patients older than 10 years, 3/0 absorbable suture was used, with six sutures positioned at 2, 4, 6, 8, 10, and 12 o'clock. The incision line was then covered with an *oxytetracycline* hydrochloride-*Polymyxin B sulfate* antibiotic combination containing a bandage. It affects by preventing the bacteria's cell wall and the labor of the bacteria's proteins. Patients were observed for 2 h postoperatively and analgesics were prescribed before discharge. The first follow-up was performed by the operating team, and 10 days after the operation, the wound dressing was removed in the Pediatric Surgery Outpatient Clinic, and a return to daily life was recommended.

Afterward, the patients and their parents were advised to continue their daily life routines. In cases of excoriation due to phimosis, the application of epithelizing cream to the wound was recommended to the patient or his family. Possible complications were explained to patients and parents, and we asked them to visit the hospital if they developed any symptoms, such as penile bleeding, discoloration, or shape changes. In these cases, patients were measured, followed, and treated by the first author of this article.

They were not given oral antibiotics to use prophylactically or at home. We recommend ibuprofen to children as an anti-inflammatory analgesic 5–7 mg/kg after 1 year old and paracetamol 10–15 mg/kg before 1 year old every 8 h.

The perioperative complications group included bleeding during the circumcision or during the hospital stay. The early postoperative complications group emerged during the first 10 days after discharge from the hospital. The long-term complications group occurred in 10 or more days after discharge from the hospital. The complications related to the circumcisions were assessed with the modified Clavien-Dindo classification system [12].

The following symptoms were not measured as complications: foreskin swelling, glans penis incrustation due to a phimosis opening, or a temporary color change after local anesthesia.

3. Statistical analysis

The investigation set consisting of those patients circumcised using the thermocautery-assisted method was measured with the Statistical Package for the Social Sciences software (SPSS Inc., Chicago, IL, USA). The output dispersion was examined using the Kolmogorov-Smirnov test. The continuous variables were expressed as the mean ± standard deviation (range: minimum-maximum), and the appropriate categorical variables were indicated as the numbers and percentages. The chi-squared and Mann-Whitney U tests were referred to measure the categorical output and the quantitative changeable, respectively. Two-tailed P values of less than 0.05 were accepted as statistically substantial.

4. Results

The mean age of the patients was 4.89 ± 2.08 years (range: 50 days to 17 years). The average surgical duration was 7.484 ± 1.524 min (range: 5–20 min). The complication rates for the age groups of the patients included in the study were as follows: 30 days to 6 months: 2 (0.3%), 6–12 months: 17 (4.7%), 1–3 years: 22 (14.4%), 3–6 years: 10 (18.5%), and 6–17 years: 2 (0.3%). Complications were observed in 53 patients or 2.9% of the whole dataset. The complications were assessed with the modified Clavien-Dindo classification method. Two (0.11%) of the patients had bleeding from the suture line, which was classified as a perioperative complication. The bleedings were stopped immediately via cauterization. Twenty-eight (1.54%) of the patients who underwent circumcision had postoperative early complications. Eight (0.44%) infections and 12 (0.66%) bleeding cases were classified as early postoperative early complications. The infection was treated with antibiotics and dressing.

Due to a ligated artery, a 4-year-old patient had frenular artery bleeding on the first day after the circumcision, and it was controlled after taking to the operating room and opening the sutures with local anesthesia. Five of all patients who underwent circumcision bleeding were controlled by stitching up also with local anesthesia. Their ages were 11 months, 22 months, 3 years, 4 years, and 5.5 years, respectively. Six of all patients had dorsal vein bleeding treated via vein ligation also with local anesthesia. Their ages were 10 months, 16 months, 18 months, 22 months, 3 years, and 4 years, respectively.

Seven (0.38%) of all patients developed convulsions due to local anesthesia. Their ages were 8 months, 9 months, 10 months, 10 months, 1 year, 1 year, and 1 year, respectively. Four of these convulsions were as nystagmus form and three were in the tonic-clonic form. The reason for the high number of convulsions under 1 year of age may be allergy to bupivacaine. All the convulsions were followed by rectal diazepam (0.5 mg/kg) for 24 h. In one case (0.05%), a 2.5-year-old patient could not urinate for the first 8 h after local anesthesia, but this patient urinated spontaneously without a urinary catheter. Twenty-three (1.26%) of the patients who underwent circumcision had late complications. The penises of two patients were trapped, and they were surgically circumcised again. A total of five patients aged 7, 10, 12, 17, and 21 months during the circumcision required urethral dilatations after 1 month because of the meatal stenosis. A 1-year-old patient developed meatitis 10 days after the circumcision, while a 2-year-old patient had the same issue 1 month after the circumcision. Both children were medically treated.

Epidermal granuloma and inclusion cysts in the dorsal or ventral part of the penis were removed from the suture line with local anesthesia in four (0.22%) cases. Their ages of them were 4 months, 9 months, 14 months, and 2.5 years, respectively. After circumcision, six of seven (0.38%) cases where the mucosa adhered were opened by simply retracting, while the skin bridge in one case was cut with a scalpel under local anesthesia. Although we coagulated the vessels by holding them one by one, we saw ecchymotic changes in the skin in one case after circumcision and lacerations due to a burn at the edge of the skin during the procedure in three cases. There was no problem with the follow-up. Finally, one patient had a glans-skin bridge complication 6 months after the circumcision, and he was treated surgically.

Secondary phimosis was detected in four (0.21%) of our cases, and they were treated with circumcision revision. Their ages were 10 months, 14 months, 1.5 years, and 2 years, respectively.

Urethral injury and fistula occurred in a 4-year-old patient with a urethral ventral chord. About 1 year later, urethral fistula repair was performed under general anesthesia.

Except for four patients, complications were only observed in children older than 6 months and younger than 6 years old. The patients younger than 6 months and older than 6 years had significantly lower complication rates when compared to the other patients, and this comparison was statistically significant (P = 0.001).

5. Discussion

Circumcision has been done as a routine for all recently born males in Muslim countries. Circumcision keeps on be done for religious, cultural, and medical reasons. The prevalence of circumcision in the United States is predicted to be about 80% for males, with most of these procedures carried out in newborns [13].

A recent meta-analysis comprised 140 journal articles that came to the same outcome; early infant male circumcision has long-standing advantages. It was shown to protect against urinary tract infections, phimosis, inflammatory skin conditions, candidiasis, various sexually transmitted diseases (STDs) in both sexes, genital ulcers, and penile, prostate, and cervical cancer [14]. Unfavorable effects of circumcisions are uncommon. The low risk in comparison to the benefit demonstrates that the benefits of male circumcision surpass its risk. Adverse events of circumcision have been difficult to measure accurately. The largest studies on measuring complication rates are mostly retrospective, and their data have generally not taken into account standardizing the variables. The timing of the procedure, the technique, the person performing the procedure, the setting, and the equipment used can all change the percentage of overall complications significantly.

Male circumcision has a low incidence of unfavorable events overall, particularly if the procedure was performed during the first year of life [15]. The risk is further decreased and might be prevented, with careful consideration of the penile anatomy and the correct use of surgical equipment by trained clinicians in sterile environments. Most of the unfavorable events of circumcision are mild and are easily treatable. Although there are different plots of the diverse circumcision methods in the literature, researchers are still negotiating the most available circumcision age and the reliable circumcision method. The applied technique should be applicable, common, and reliable, and it should cause very few or no challenges. For this purpose, we compared the thermocautery-assisted method with the other circumcision methods in terms of the early and long-term complications. The early complications included bleeding, pain, inadequate skin removal, infection, chordee, iatrogenic hypospadias, glanular necrosis, and glanular amputation. The long-term complications included epidermal inclusion cysts, suture sinus, penile adhesions, phimosis, urethrocutaneous fistula, trapped penis, meatitis, and meatal stenosis [7, 16, 17]. In addition, hydronephrosis and permanent renal damage can be caused by meatal stenosis [18]. In our study, we did not see hydronephrosis and permanent renal damage caused by meatal stenosis.

The thermocautery-assisted technique utilizes the heat energy used for cauterizing. When compared with the monopolar cautery technique, which utilize an electrical current, the thermocautery-assisted method conducts the heat locally. According to the skin features of the patient, the heat levels are adaptable on the most recently developed thermocautery devices. Former studies have shown that optimum hemostasis is accomplished with a temperature ranging between 100°C and 400°C. Although a range between 350°C and 900°C can be obtained within in vivo environments, the highest heat level is reduced by half in a bloody environment. Thermocautery devices have been used successfully in local dermatological excisions with the implementation of cardiac devices [19]. However, there have been few studies on the use of thermocauterization in circumcisions [20–23]. It has been declared that the thermocautery technique results in alike wound healing when compared to the scalpel technique [22].

Aslan et al. performed mass circumcisions with thermocautery devices in Sudan, and they reported a complication rate of 0.086% in the early postsurgical period (3 weeks). These complications included bleeding, scrotal abscess, tachycardia, and syncope after the local anesthesia injection. Up to the present moment, few data on thermocautery-assisted circumcision have been marked. However, in the study by Arslan et al., edema appeared in one-fifth of patients, which was identified as clinically inconsiderable [20]. Kazem et al. performed 3-min manual frenular compressions for bleeding control in 3760 newborn patients undergoing Plastibell circumcisions. They also used an ophthalmological thermocautery technique on a different study set including 3750 patients. While a 0.5% complication rate was observed in the first group, the thermocautery method exhibited a 0.05% complication rate [24]. Although urinary retention has been reported when using the Plastibell technique, the ophthalmological thermocautery-assisted circumcisions took longer with regard to urinary retention and wound healing [24, 25].

There are many different circumcision techniques currently in use. For example, the Plastibell circumcision technique can be applied safely in infants from newborns to 1 year olds [26]. The operation takes between 5 and 10 min, and the Plastibell is abandoned in the penis for 1 or 2 weeks until it comes off by itself. Complications related to this method have been reported in 3% of the patients [26], and Jimoh et al. reported a complication rate of 1.1% in their Plastibell study of 2276 patients [27]. The Mogen clamp is often used among the Jewish population [28], and Young et al. reported a complication rate of 2.7% in their Mogen clamp study of 1239 patients [29]. Ali's clamp is a tool widely used in Turkey. It consists of a whistle-shaped tube on the glans and a ring that compresses the foreskin through it. The average duration of this application is approximately 5 min. Senel et al. reported a complication rate of 2% in their Ali's clamp study of 7500 patients [30]. They showed that Ali's clamp is easier to apply, and the operation time was less than in the other current methods, with fewer complications [30]. Another technique uses the Shang ring, which was developed in China. It is an apparatus that compresses the foreskin between two rings; however, this method carries the risk of glans amputation [31]. The ring is removed after 5–7 days [32]. In one meta-analysis including 18 randomized clinical studies, Huang et al. reported a complication rate of 1.27% in 2589 patients circumcised using Shang rings [33] The Gomco method uses a metal clamp with a bell-shaped tip, and Amir et al. reported a complication rate of 1.9% in their study of 1000 patients [34]. Ozen et al. reported that 13 newborns who were circumcised using the Gomco technique developed meatal stenoses. Meatoplasties were used to treat these patients [17].

The dorsal slit, guillotine, and sleeve methods are defined as open circumcision surgical techniques. For the dorsal slit method, a vertical incision is made in the forward direction; then, an appropriate amount of mucosa is selected with the foreskin and removed by cutting the tissue around the penis with scissors. Following hemostasis, the remaining skin and mucosa are stitched together. In the sleeve technique, the incision on the foreskin is done circularly with a scalpel, and the mucosal boundaries are excised. The skin is cut in the form of a band and then removed. This process is followed by hemostasis and stitching. Buwembo et al. reported a complication rate of 0.6% in their dorsal slit study of 2471 patients and a complication rate of 1.4% in their sleeve study of 2681 patients [35]. The application of monopolar diathermy runs the potential risk of coagulation due to the electrical current at the penile base. Previous studies have revealed serious complications, such as penile ablation, necrosis, and gangrene [36]. Shen et al. compared two disposable circumcision suture devices (Langhe and Daming). Complications such as bleeding, manual staple removal, and infections are frequently observed when using these devices [37]. Seven (0.38%) of all patients developed convulsions due to local anesthesia. Four of these were as nystagmus form and three were as the tonic-clonic form. The reason for the high number of convulsions under 1 year of age may be an allergy to bupivacaine. In one case (0.05%), a 2.5-year-old patient could not urinate for the first 8 h after local anesthesia, but this patient urinated spontaneously without a urinary catheter. Our observations show that children under 6 months and over 6 years of age have fewer short- and long-term complications when undergoing circumcisions. In our study, the complication rate was 2.9% in 1821 patients. The fact that the complication rates of circumcisions performed under 6 months and over 6 years of age are similar to the literature makes us think that this procedure with local anesthesia is especially more reliable in this age group in children. In a study carried out in England, 66,519 circumcisions were reported, with a complication rate of 2%. Complications were hemorrhage in 533 patients (0.8%), need for a revision in 303 patients (0.5%), and meatal stenosis in seven patients [38]. In the present study, similar to the literature, the most common early circumcision complication was found to be bleeding (0.77% of 1821 patients).

According to our observations, the circumcision line usually heals within 5 days before 6 months and 7 days after 6 months when using the thermocautery technique. We observed that the wound healing was extended to 20 days in only two patients in our data set. Their ages are 8 and 10 years old during the circumcision. In addition, urinary retention was observed in one patient in our thermocautery-assisted circumcisions.

6. Conclusion

According to our observations, the circumcision line usually heals within 10 days under 6 months of age when using the thermocautery technique. We observed that the wound healing was extended by 3 weeks in five patients in our data set, but their circumcision ages were over 1 year. Our observations show that children under 6 months and over 6 years of age have fewer short- and long-term complications when undergoing circumcisions. This chapter provides a complete evaluation of the thermocautery-assisted circumcision technique with respect to the short- and long-term complications. The patients in our dataset were followed up postoperatively for 1 month to 1 year. Since the cauterization is performed during the cutting process in the thermocautery technique, the bleeding risk is less when compared to the other methods. In recent years, in Turkey, circumcisions have been increasingly preferred for children at earlier ages, due to the belief that this leads to faster wound healing.

Urethral injury and fistula occurred in a 4-year-old patient with a urethral ventral chord. His urethral plate was very thin and weak, so urethracutaneous fistula occurred. About 1 year later, urethral fistula repair was performed under general anesthesia. The prolongation of postoperative discharge time after general anesthesia often causes pain, nausea, and vomiting. No nausea and vomiting were observed in our cases. All our patients were discharged on the day of the operation. For adequate sedation, anxiolysis, and analgesia in circumcision cases, a safe perioperative process should be planned.

The main advantages of this technique are the cheap cost, the ability to heal the tissue in a short time, and the ability to perform it in a nonoperating room environment with local anesthesia by a specialist doctor. This can be done fairly quickly and allows for much more circumcision in all the age groups of children in areas where the cost and availability of general anesthesia are prohibited.

As a result, this technique reveals that it is a safe, practical, reliable, and effective method for performing circumcisions in children, especially under 6 months and over 6 years of age.

Conflict of interest/funding

None.

Author details

Mehmet Uysal
Department of Pediatric Surgery, Karamanoğlu Mehmetbey University School of Medicine, Karaman, Turkey

*Address all correspondence to: drmyzuysal3@gmail.com

References

[1] Rudolph C, Rudolph A, Lister G, First L, Gershon A. McGraw-Hill Companies, Inc. Vol. 188. 2016. p. 978

[2] Lerman SE, Liao JC. Neonatal circumcision. Pediatric Clinic. 2001;**48**(6):1539-1557

[3] Holman JR, Lewis EL. Neonatal circumcision techniques. American Family Physician. 1995;**52**:511-518

[4] Niku SD, Stock JA, Kaplan GW. Neonatal circumcision. Urologic Clinics of North America. 1995;**22**(1):57-65

[5] Rizvi SAH, Naqvi SAA, Hussain M, Hasan AS. Religious circumcision: A Muslim view. BJU International. 1999;**83**(suppl. 1):13-16

[6] Prabhakaran S, Ljuhar D, Coleman R, Nataraja RM. Circumcision in the paediatric patient: A review of indications, technique and complications. Journal of Paediatrics and Child Health. 2018;**54**:1299-1307

[7] Krill AJ, Palmer LS, Palmer JS. Complications of circumcision. Scientific World Journal. 2011;**11**:2458-2468

[8] Weiss HA, Larke N, Halperin D, Schenker I. Complications of circumcision in male neonates, infants and children: A systematic review. BMC Urology. 2010;**10**:2

[9] Morris BJ, Wamai RG, Henebeng EB, Tobian AA, Klausner JD, Banerjee J, et al. Estimation of countryspecific and global prevalence of male circumcision. Population Health Metrics. 2016;**14**:4

[10] American Academy of Pediatrics. Circumcision policy statement. Pediatrics. 2012;**130**:585-586

[11] Thorup J, Thorup SC, Ifaoui IB. Complication rate after circumcision in a paediatric surgical setting should not be neglected. Danish Medical Journal. 2013;**60**(8):A4681

[12] Clavien PA, Barkun J, de Oliveira ML, et al. The Clavien-Dindo classification of surgical complications: Five-year experience. Annals of Surgery. 2009;**250**:187-196

[13] Introcaso CE, Xu F, Kilmarx PH, Zaidi A, Markowitz LE. Prevalence of circumcision among men and boys aged 14 to 59 years in the United States, National Health and nutrition examination surveys 2005-2010. Sexually Transmitted Diseases. 2013;**40**(7):521-525

[14] Morris BJ, Kennedy SE, Wodak AD, Mindel A, Golovsky D, Schrieber L, et al. Early infant male circumcision: Systematic review, risk-benefit analysis, and progress in policy. World Journal of Clinical Pediatrics. 2017;**6**(1):89-102

[15] El Bcheraoui C, Zhang X, Cooper CS, Rose CE, Kilmarx PH, Chen RT. Rates of adverse events associated with male circumcision in U.S. medical settings, 2001 to 2010. JAMA Pediatrics. 2014;**168**(7):625-634

[16] Eke N. Major surgical complications from minor urological procedures. Journal of the National Medical Association. 2000;**2000**(92):196-199

[17] Özen MA, Gündoğdu G, Taşdemir M, Eroğlu E. Complication of newborn circumcision: Meatal stenosis or meatal web? Journal of Pediatric Urology. 2017. DOI: 10.1016/j.jpurol.2017.05.007

[18] Saeedi P, Ahmadnia H, Akhavan RA. Evaluation of the effect of meatal

stenosis on the urinary tract by using ultrasonography. Urology Journal. 2017;**14**:3071-3074

[19] Lane JE, O'Brien EM, Kent DE. Optimization of thermocautery in excisional dermatologic surgery. Dermatologic Surgery. 2006;**32**:669-675

[20] Arslan D, Kalkan M, Yazgan H, Unuvar U, Şahin C. Collective circumcision performed in Sudan: Evaluation in terms of early complications and alternative practice. Urology. 2013;**81**:864-868

[21] Abdel HS. The use of thermal cautery for male circumcision. JKAU Medical Science. 2009;**16**:89-93

[22] Tuncer AA, Bozkurt MF, Bayraktaroğlu A, et al. Examination of histopathological changes of scalpel, monopolar, bipolar, and thermocautery applications in rat experimental circumcision model. American Journal of Translational Research. 2017;**9**:2306-2313

[23] Karaman MI, Zulfikar B, Caskurlu T, Ergenekon E. Circumcision in hemophilia: A cost-effective method using a novel device. Journal of Pediatric Surgery. 2004;**39**:1562-1564

[24] Kazeem MM, Mehdi AZ, Golrasteh KZ, Behzad FZ. Comparative evaluation of two techniques of hemostasis in neonatal circumcision using the Plastibell® device. Journal of Pediatric Urology. 2010;**6**:258-260

[25] Mihssin N, Moorthy K, Houghton WJ. Retention of urine: An unusual complication of the Plastibell device. BJU International. 1999;**84**:747

[26] Moosa FA, Khan FW, Rao MH. Comparison of complications of circumcision by 'Plastibell device technique' in male neonates and infants. The Journal of the Pakistan Medical Association. 2010;**60**:664-667

[27] Jimoh BM, Odunayo IS, Chinwe I, Akinfolarin OO, Oluwafemi A, Olusanmi EJ. Plastibell circumcision of 2,276 male infants: A multi-Centre study. The Pan African Medical Journal. 2016:23-35

[28] Reynolds RD. Use of the Mogen clamp for neonatal circumcision. American Family Physician. 1996;**54**:177-182

[29] Young MR, Bailey RC, Odoyo-June E, et al. Safety of over twelve hundred infant male circumcisions using the Mogen clamp in Kenya. PLoS One. 2012;**7**:47395

[30] Senel FM, Demirelli M, Oztek S. Minimally invasive circumcision with a novel plastic clamp technique: A review of 7,500 cases. Pediatric Surgery International. 2010;**26**:739-745

[31] Abdulwahab-Ahmed A, Mungadi IA. Techniques of male circumcision. Journal of Surgical Technique Case Report. 2013;**5**:1-7

[32] Awori QD, Lee RK, Li PS, et al. Use of the Shang ring circumcision device in boys below 18 years old in Kenya: Results from a pilot study. Journal of the International AIDS Society. 2017;**20**:1-8

[33] Huang C, Song P, Xu C, Wang R, Wei L, Zhao X. Comparative efficacy and safety of different circumcisions for patients with redundant prepuce or phimosis: A network meta-analysis. International Journal of Surgery. 2017;**43**:17-25

[34] Amir M, Raja MH, Niaz WA. Neonatal circumcision with Gomco clamp--a hospital-based retrospective study of 1000 cases. The Journal of

the Pakistan Medical Association. 2000;**50**:224-227

[35] Buwembo DR, Musoke R, Kigozi G, et al. Evaluation of the safety and efficiency of the dorsal slit and sleeve methods of male circumcision provided by physicians and clinical officers in Rakai, Uganda. BJU International. 2012;**109**:104-108

[36] Uzun G, Ozdemir Y, Eroglu M, Mutluoglu M. Electrocautery-induced gangrene of the glans penis in a child following circumcision. BML Case Reports. 2012

[37] Shen J, Shi J, Gao J, et al. A comparative study on the clinical efficacy of two different disposable circumcision suture devices in adult males. Urology Journal. 2017;**14**:5013-5017

[38] Cathcart P, Nuttall M, Meulen JV, et al. Trends in paediatric circumcision and its complications in England between 1997 and 2003. The British Journal of Surgery. 2003;**93**:885-890